THE Medicare ANSWER BOOK

Connacht Cash

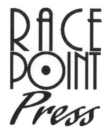

RACE POINT *Press*

The Medicare Answer Book © 1998 by Connacht Cash

Published by Race Point Press
15 Standish Way, P.O. Box 770
Provincetown, MA 02657-0770
(508) 487-1626 ■ info@RacePointPress.com

This book was written to provide basic information on the subject of Medicare. The information provided is based on the experience of the author, with the understanding that the author is not engaged in rendering legal or other professional services herein.

This text should be used as a general guide and readers should consult with appropriate counsel regarding specific financial or legal questions. Every effort has been made to make this text as accurate as possible. Neither the author nor the publisher accepts any responsibility with respect to any loss or damage caused, or alleged to be caused, by errors, omissions, or misinterpretation of the information provided.

Cover Design: Mike Wright
Author Photograph: Joel Brodsky
Book Design: Sara Patton

Printed in the United States
1 3 5 7 9 10 8 6 4 2

Publisher's Cataloging-in-Publication
(Provided by Quality Books, Inc.)

Cash, Connacht.
    The Medicare answer book / by Connacht Cash.—2nd ed.
    p. cm.
    Includes index.
    Preassigned LCCN: 98-65682
    ISBN: 0-9633145-4-8 (pbk.)

    1. Medicare. 2. Aged—Medical care—United States. I. Title.

HD7102.U4C38 1998   368.4'26'00973
                             QBI98-500

Table of Contents

Preface

So, why should I care about Medicare?

My own answer is actually quite simple. Both of my parents were covered by Medicare during retirement and they were affected by Medicare's coverage, or lack of it, for over twenty years. In assisting them, I learned firsthand what Medicare is all about for seniors—and for their family members who are called upon to help. I also learned how severe the financial consequences of Medicare's gaps can be.

Emotional crises often seem to propel us in new directions. The first edition of this book was the result of such a situation. The emotional roller coaster of dealing with my parents' illnesses was complicated by Medicare and, in their memory, I intend to do what I can so that this burden is lightened for others. I can't rework the system (heaven help us all, the politicians are in control there) but hopefully I can help people to understand it better and navigate it successfully.

Medicare is a godsend for millions of people because it allows them to have medical insurance without regard to health status. But Medicare is not perfect. This is a well intentioned and very necessary program that is poorly understood, difficult to navigate and needlessly complicated.

Life seems to get busier and more complicated daily for everyone I know. This book is my attempt to make one area less complicated. I fervently hope that my effort will help other families to understand what Medicare really covers—

and to avoid the risks to their peace of mind and their finances that lack of such knowledge can bring.

In closing I also want to urge my fellow baby boomers *to find out now* how Medicare works—before they need to know about it to help a family member. At the very least, I strongly suggest that families discuss what insurance coverage exists and what to do in the event of an emergency. Believe me, the paperwork is the last thing you want to deal with when illness strikes.

Introduction

This book will take the mystery out of Medicare and will help folks who aren't in the insurance business to understand what it covers and what it doesn't—and how to protect themselves from unforeseen financial disaster.

Medicare covers over 38 million people and it is assumed to be very comprehensive coverage. Well, it is and it isn't. And what you know or don't know about Medicare can affect what kind of treatment is received, where it is given, and for how long it continues.

The most widespread misperception about Medicare is that it will pay for long-term care. *It doesn't.* Another is that continuing coverage for medical care is basically unlimited. *It isn't.* Yet another is that all doctors accept what Medicare considers a reasonable charge for their services. *Not true.*

All health care insurance policies have limitations and requirements that must be met for receiving reimbursement. The same is true of Medicare. It also has deductibles, co-payments, and items it simply does not pay for, such as prescriptions.

Dealing with insurance is not usually high on anyone's list of fun things to do. And since it often seems to be arbitrary in nature and always requires sorting through confusing documents, many people try to ignore it until, unfortunately, they need it.

To properly understand Medicare, this book will make the following areas user friendly:

- The language
- The forms
- The types of coverage available
- The "how to" of deciding what additional coverage you need to have
- The questions you need to ask
- The way to challenge a decision you believe is wrong
- The way to keep track of your claims, so you don't pay for something you don't owe

You will see examples of how Medicare works, how it doesn't work, and get answers to many frequently asked questions. The new options will be discussed, as well as how to make sense of these choices.

Since its inception, the Medicare program has been difficult to understand, and coverage choices were limited. The Balanced Budget Act of 1997 added new and very different choices to the Medicare menu. Traditional fee-for-service Medicare still exists, but now there are new and varied options for managed care and for catastrophic care plans. So you have more choices, but the explanations are just as fuzzy.

The rapid and continuing increases in the cost of medical care require that we all be well-informed consumers. For Medicare beneficiaries and their families, this means making reasoned judgments about sensible ways to protect themselves from the potential financial disaster of large, unanticipated medical bills.

There is no reason that anyone should pay more than s/he is legally required to, but many people do because they are confused about their obligations. By the end of this book, you'll know the options for filling in the gaps in Medicare's coverage and what your exposure to costs really is. This book will help you to become a better informed Medicare consumer.

By learning what kinds of decisions should be made now— before someone is surprised and left with a financial burden— you protect yourself and your family. In the best of all possible worlds, you will have the information and never need it.

But, isn't it always better to be prepared?

SECTION I
MEDICARE, MEDIGAP, MEDI-WHAT?

Medicare, Medigap and Medicaid

Medicare

Medicare has been around since the mid-1960s. As one of the so-called "Great Society" programs, which were enacted with a great deal of good will and not a lot of thought about how to pay for them, Medicare was added to the Social Security Act in 1965. Generally thought of as medical care for the elderly, it also covers four million disabled people.

Of all the Great Society programs, Medicare is arguably, one of the most successful. Intended to help protect the elderly by ensuring that they can get medical insurance coverage at an affordable rate after age 65, Medicare provides something the private sector cannot be relied upon to provide.

Medicare has accomplished two things: coverage is available without regard to medical condition and at the same price for everyone based on uniform eligibility requirements. This makes the program unique. These are both important points, as those of us who have ever tried to get insurance after a major illness or with a less than ideal medical history understand.

In the 1970s, responsibility for administering the Medicare program was given to the Health Care Financing Agency

(HCFA). In what was viewed as a streamlining measure, this agency was given control of several government medical care programs, including Medicare and Medicaid.

HCFA's mission is to control health care costs associated with the programs assigned to it. The agency makes the rules and regulations which standardize payments for services, defines what type of care is reasonable for various health care needs, and supervises the certification of Medicare providers.

HCFA effectively controls all Medicare operations, from the amount paid to a doctor or hospital to deciding which HMO plan will be available in your area. The net effect on Medicare beneficiaries is that a surprising number of non-medical personnel are in a position to second-guess a doctor's treatment plan. This increases the need to be a well-informed Medicare consumer.

The Future

The number of people enrolled in the Medicare program has increased by 93 percent since it began. By 1997, Medicare covered 38 million people, about 15 percent of the population. As we proceed into the twenty-first century and the population ages, these numbers will soar, thanks to improvements in health care techniques and increases in longevity. The Census Bureau currently predicts that 20 percent of the population will be 65 or older by 2030—an estimated 70 million people who will be eligible for Medicare.

We'll live longer, but the odds are that our health will still deteriorate with age. In 1993, older people accounted for 36 percent of all hospital stays. That means that we all face the possibility of some substantial medical bills while covered by Medicare. It seems practical to make certain that we each

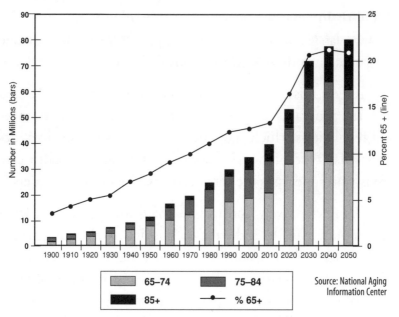

Growth of the 65+ Population, by Age Group: 1900 to 2050

understand exactly what Medicare covers now (and keep an eye on the changes proposed for the future) so that we can protect ourselves and our loved ones from the financial quicksand that can be associated with medical bills. So let's start with the basics.

Medicare, Medigap, and Medicaid

Before discussing the ins and outs of Medicare, we need to clear up the confusion associated with three terms that sound alike, but are very different.

Medicare, Medigap, and Medicaid can all be involved in paying for medical bills, but they are separate and distinct in their application. The first two programs work together and are for financially independent people; the last one aids people who have exhausted their financial resources almost entirely.

◤ *Medicare*

This health insurance program is funded by the federal government from payroll tax contributions and general tax revenues. There are three "Parts" to Medicare—Part A, Part B and Part C (Part C is new in 1998).

Part A (Medicare Hospital Insurance) and Part B (Medicare Medical Insurance) combine to form what most people think of as Medicare. They are the traditional fee-for-service Medicare plan, in which a patient has free choice as to medical care.

Part A and Part B each cover very different types of medical expenses, and they will be discussed in greater detail in later chapters. You can enroll in either Part A or Part B, or you can have both. The premium for Part B is deducted from your Social Security check monthly, while Part A doesn't cost you anything once you are eligible.

(For consistency, we will refer to them as Part A and Part B throughout the book, as that is the most common way that you will hear them used.)

Part C (Medicare+Choice) is the new section of Medicare created by the Balanced Budget Act of 1997. All of Medicare's managed care options (e.g., HMOs) will be consolidated under Part C by 1999. If you opt for coverage under Part C, you will not need coverage under Part A or Part B. Eligibility for Part C coverage is the same as for Part A and Part B and your premium will be the same as that charged for Part B coverage.

In addition to its managed care options, Part C will also include some plans which are targeted to more affluent Medicare beneficiaries: Medical Savings Accounts (MSAs) and *Private* Fee-for-Service plans. MSAs are designed for people who prefer to buy catastrophic care coverage and can afford the financial risk involved. Private Fee-for-Service plans will be allowed to set their own fee schedules for participating doctors and patients, rather than adhering to Medicare's approved amounts. We'll discuss these new options in more detail in later chapters.

◤ Medigap

This term refers to insurance policies that are sold by private insurance companies. These policies are designed to supplement, or fill the gaps in, Medicare Part A and Part B coverage by paying for expenses that would otherwise be paid out of your own funds. (You will not need a Medigap policy if you have Part C managed care coverage.)

Medigap policies are not government sponsored, but they are regulated as to form and content to make it easier for consumers to compare pricing. The standard policies are labeled A – J and there is a wide range in coverage between the least expensive policy type (Policy A) and the most comprehensive one (Policy J).

◤ Medicaid

This is a government program that helps people with little or no financial resources of their own. The federal government contributes funding for Medicaid, but the states set the rules and regulations for coverage. Therefore, they vary from state to state.

Medicaid is often confused with Medicare because many *Medicaid* patients are elderly and in nursing homes. Unlike Medicare, eligibility for Medicaid is based on financial need. Unfortunately, many elderly long-term care patients end up using this program because their resources have been exhausted by medical expenses not covered by Medicare or other insurance.

Medicaid eligibility and coverage varies from state to state within federal guidelines.

Each of these different programs will be discussed in greater detail later in the book.

Frequently Asked Questions

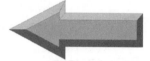

Q. What is Medicare?

A. Medicare is a federal health insurance program covering those 65 years or older, the disabled, and people with permanent renal failure. It is administered by the Health Care Financing Administration (HCFA) of the U.S. Department of Health and Human Services.

Q. How is Medicare financed?

A. Medicare is financed from the Social Security payroll tax collected from employees and employers, from the self-employment tax paid by individuals, and from general tax revenues. In addition, 25 percent of the cost of Medicare Part B coverage is financed by the monthly premiums paid by beneficiaries ($43.80 per month in 1998).

Q. What does Social Security have to do with Medicare?

A. Eligibility for Medicare is calculated on a basis similar to that of Social Security eligibility. If you are eligible for Social Security payments, you are eligible for Medicare. You can get information about Medicare and enroll in the program at your local Social Security office. Information is available from the Social Security Administration by calling (800) 772-1213.

Q. I have Medicare; how can I tell if it is Part A or Part B?

A. Look on your Medicare identification card. On the lower half of the card, it will list which coverage you have and the effective date(s) of the coverage.

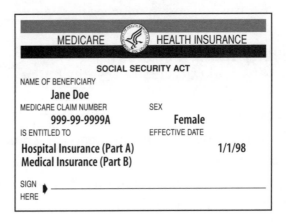

Q. How do I get a Medigap policy?

A. Medigap policies are sold by private insurance companies. Call your state insurance office for a list of the companies that are licensed to sell Medigap policies in your state. There is a list of state insurance departments in Appendix D.

Q. What is HCFA?

A. HCFA stands for the Health Care Financing Administration. This federal agency is responsible for administering the Medicare program and setting the standards used for evaluating claims and payments.

Q. Is it possible to have Medicare coverage and also be in the Medicaid program?

A. Yes. If you are covered by both programs, charges for medical treatment will be submitted for payment to Medicare first.

Q. There is a letter after the Medicare claim number on my card. What is it for?

A. It is a code used by Social Security to indicate the type of benefits you are receiving. Always include the letters on all Medicare forms and correspondence.

Q. How does Medicaid affect the elderly?

A. Most Medicaid dollars are spent paying for nursing home care for the elderly. Contrary to popular belief, Medicare does not pay for nursing home care and many nursing home residents exhaust their financial resources after being admitted to a nursing home. Medicaid often pays for this long-term care.

Q. How do I get information about Medicaid programs?

A. Contact your state's Medicaid office. A complete list is provided in Appendix E.

Q. Where can I get a list of Medigap carriers?

A. Call your state's Insurance Department (see Appendix D for contact information) and they will be able to give you a list of companies who are licensed to sell Medigap policies in your area.

Q. Are Medicare+Choice and Medicare Part C the same?

A. Yes.

Q. What kinds of plans are in Medicare Part C?

A. Included are: managed care plans, including Health Maintenance Organizations, Preferred Provider Organizations and Provider Sponsored Organizations; Medical Savings Accounts; and Private Fee-for-Service Plans (see Chapter 11).

CHAPTER 2

The Language of Medicare

<table><tr><td>Insurance Lingo—What Those Terms Really Mean</td><td>Mention the word insurance and you can easily elicit a groan from almost anyone. Whether it is about a claim that wasn't covered, or insurance company personnel giving an unintelligible answer, or about</td></tr></table>

the claim paperwork being a nightmare, it seems that everyone has some horror story about insurance.

Among the most confusing areas when dealing with insurance is understanding the language. It should be simple. And, thanks to pressure from consumer groups, most insurance contracts are written in clearer language these days. But are they really understandable?

One of the barriers to truly knowing what your insurance policy covers is that common definitions of words we use every day may not be precise enough for the clear meaning needed in an insurance policy. The insurance industry is not unique in using terms and concepts that have special meanings—all professions, trades, and industries do. The big difference is that usually we don't have to understand such words unless we are actually in that industry, profession, or trade.

When it comes to insurance, however, everyone needs to understand its unique language at some point in his/her life.

More often than not, people purchase insurance without clearly understanding what they are buying because of this lack of ready vocabulary. Sometimes words that seem perfectly understandable in everyday usage have a very narrow and specific meaning in insurance. For instance, "hospital costs" to most people would mean all the expenses related to a stay in a hospital. But in Medicare, hospital costs refer only to certain expenses which occur while a patient is in a hospital, and not to others.

Terms specific to Medicare insurance are used throughout this book, and we have included the most important ones in this chapter. An alphabetical listing in Appendix K includes these terms and others of importance. Don't give up if they seem a bit unwieldy to remember—you will eventually get used to them. The following list is not alphabetical, but is arranged in a way that makes it easier to understand the terms that follow.

Benefit Period — A Benefit Period is a time frame. Benefit Periods have beginnings and endings and affect your costs. They are used to make calculations about deductibles, co-payment amounts, and total covered costs. Part A Benefit Periods are calculated based on in-patient hospital stays and are explained in detail in Chapter 5. You can have more than one Benefit Period in a calendar year under Part A. Part B coverage does not refer specifically to Benefit Periods, but it does use the calendar year for calculating deductibles.

Actual Charge — The amount that your doctor, lab, or other medical care supplier bills to you. This is not necessarily the same as the amount that Medicare will pay. It is what the supplier or doctor believes the service or care is worth.

Approved Amount — The amount that Medicare decides the medical service or physician's care is worth. It may or may not be the same as the actual charge billed. If it is less than the actual charge, there is a limitation on how much of the difference you are responsible for paying.

Beneficiary — A Medicare beneficiary is the person who is enrolled in the Medicare program and receives the medical or other related services (i.e., the patient).

Deductible — This is the minimum amount of money for which the patient is responsible in any specific Benefit Period. Even when Medicare covers the costs of the medical expenses involved, the patient is generally responsible for an initial out-of-pocket payment. There is one deductible per Benefit Period under Part A and one deductible per calendar year under Part B.

Co-insurance — The amount of the charge (usually a percentage) that the patient is responsible for paying. This is applied against specific bills. It is sometimes referred to as the co-pay.

Assignment — This is an arrangement between Medicare and your physician or supplier in which the provider agrees to accept as full payment whatever the Medicare approved amount is. Assignment is financially beneficial to the patient, although it does not relieve the patient of responsibility for deductibles or co-insurance payments.

Inpatient — Someone who is actually admitted to a hospital or other medical facility for at least one night. Going to a hospital for a medical procedure, even a surgical one, does not mean you are an inpatient. You must stay overnight at the recommendation of your physician to be an inpatient.

Excess Charge — The difference between the Medicare approved amount and the actual charge, when the actual charge is more.

Medically Necessary — Medical services that are accepted as appropriate to the treatment of the patient's condition. To be a covered Medicare expense, the care must be deemed medically necessary. Generally, this means the treatment is usual for the illness, is required for proper care, and is provided under the guidance of a physician.

Medicare Hospital Insurance — Part A of Medicare, which covers medically necessary inpatient care in a hospital, skilled nursing facility, or psychiatric hospital. It also covers costs related to certain hospice and home health care services. Many home health care services will be shifting to Part B over the course of the next six years.

Medicare Benefits Notice — The form sent to the patient explaining how a Part A claim was handled by Medicare.

Medicare Medical Insurance — Part B of Medicare, which covers medically necessary doctor, laboratory, and other medical services not covered by Part A. Costs can be incurred in or out of a hospital.

Explanation of Medicare Benefits (EOMB) — This is the form that is sent to you telling you about your Part B claim. It details the dates and services rendered or doctors involved, the expenses Medicare will allow, what they have paid and to whom, and what your financial responsibility is. This is usually the first information you receive from Medicare about a claim.

Medicare Carrier — This is the organization (usually an insurance company) that the government uses to process Medicare

Part B claims. The information number listed on your EOMB form is that of your Medicare carrier. The companies vary by state and territory. A complete list is in Appendix A.

Medicare Intermediaries — The organizations Medicare uses to process Part A claims. A complete list by state and territory is found in Appendix A.

Fee-for-Service — This is the traditional type of medical provider/patient relationship. It simply means that the patient chooses his/her medical provider and then is billed a fee by that provider for the services rendered. This can be a doctor's fee or a fee for any other type of medical service. Under a fee-for-service arrangement, there are no restrictions about what provider you choose and you do not need to receive prior permission from anyone, unlike when using a managed care system.

Participating Physician or Supplier — A doctor or supplier who signs a yearly agreement with Medicare to accept assignment on all claims. This is helpful in reducing costs to the patient.

Outpatient — A patient who is treated at a hospital or other medical facility without being admitted to the facility overnight.

Skilled Nursing Facility (SNF) — A facility that provides skilled nursing and rehabilitation services. It may or may not be part of a hospital. It is not a nursing home.

Provider — A person (such as a doctor) or a company (such as a laboratory) that is approved to render medical or related services.

HMO or Health Maintenance Organization — An organization that acts as both the insurer and the provider of care, usually for a prepaid fee. Such organizations generally have a specific group of doctors, specialists, and other providers who must be used by the patient in order to obtain benefits.

Medicare+Choice Plans — All of the new non-traditional Medicare plan options. These include managed care plans, such as Health Maintenance Organizations (HMOs), Preferred Provider Organizations (PPOs) and Provider Sponsored Organizations (PSOs), as well as Medical Savings Accounts (MSAs) and Private Fee-for-Service (PFFS) plans. Medicare+Choice is also referred to as Part C.

Medicare Part C — The managed care and other Medicare plan options which are not the traditional fee-for-service plans. Also known as Medicare+Choice.

PPO or Preferred Provider Organization — A type of coordinated care plan, this type of organization encourages patients to use a specific group of medical providers, but does not require it. The plans encourage members to use network providers by making it more financially advantageous to do so. Generally, the patient pays a greater portion of the cost if the patient uses someone outside the list of approved providers and has little or no cost when using someone in the plan. This is a type of Medicare+Choice plan.

Indemnity Health Insurance Plan — Insurance that reimburses on a fee-for-service basis without restrictions on choice of doctors, hospitals, etc. Traditional Medicare coverage is a type of indemnity plan.

Managed Care — This is a medical care delivery system, such as an HMO or PPO, where someone "manages" your care by making decisions regarding which medical services you can use. Each plan has its own group of hospitals, doctors, and other providers and you generally must receive all your care through someone in this network. The benefits of managed care plans are that they often cover preventive care and do not usually require you to fill out any paperwork. These plans may require a co-payment. Managed care plans may charge you an additional monthly fee for services provided that are not typical of Medicare coverage.

Coordinated Care — The same as Managed Care.

Medical Savings Account (MSAs) — A high deductible ($6000) medical insurance plan. These plans will be available to a limited number of beneficiaries beginning in 1999 so that HCFA can evaluate their effectiveness. They are a Medicare+Choice program.

Provider Sponsored Organizations (PSOs) — Another type of coordinated care plan. This is a public or private entity organized by a group of health care providers that provides a substantial proportion of health care services directly to beneficiaries. This is a type of Medicare+Choice plan.

Primary Payer — The primary payer, usually Medicare, is the party with the first responsibility for payment of a bill for medical services. You may have secondary payers, such as Medigap policies, that will require submittal of the bill after processing by the primary payer. Under some circumstances, Medicare is not the primary payer, for example if you are covered by an employer-sponsored health care plan. It is very important to understand who the primary payer is, as it affects your paperwork and your reimbursement.

Secondary Payer — The party (insurance company or Medicare) that is responsible for payments after the primary payer has processed the claim. If you are covered by an employer-sponsored group health care plan, Medicare will be the secondary payer.

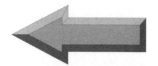

Frequently Asked Questions

Q. I received several notifications of claim payments from Medicare after a recent inpatient hospital visit. Why are there two different numbers to call for information?

A. The claim for costs covered by Medicare Part A was processed by the Medicare intermediary in your state. The claim for Medicare Part B costs was handled by the Medicare carrier in your state. They can be, but are not always, the same organization. Also, Part A and Part B costs are handled separately for payment, so you will always receive separate notices.

Q. I am covered under my company's health insurance plan and I have Medicare coverage. I received an EOMB form for a doctor's visit and Medicare did not pay the costs. Why?

A. If you are covered by an employer's plan, Medicare is the secondary payer. You need to submit the doctor's bill to your employer's plan first. If there is a balance due after it is processed, the remainder should be submitted to Medicare for payment.

Q. What is an EOMB form?

A. The initials stand for Explanation of Medicare Benefits. When a Part B claim is submitted to Medicare, you will receive an EOMB form detailing how much Medicare paid on your behalf and how much you are responsible for paying.

Q. What is an actual charge?

A. The amount billed to you by your doctor, hospital, lab, or other medical supplier for services rendered.

Q. What is the difference between an actual charge and an approved charge?

A. The actual charge is the amount billed to you by the medical provider. The approved charge is the amount Medicare determines it will pay for the service provided to you. If the approved amount is less than the actual charge, you will be responsible for some or all of the difference unless the provider has accepted assignment. If you have other insurance coverage you should submit the claim to the secondary payer for additional payment.

Q. Why is it beneficial to me for my doctor to be a participating physician?

A. It can save you money because participating physicians accept the amount that Medicare decides is the appropriate payment (approved amount) for their services. You will still be responsible for deductibles and co-payments, but your exposure to out-of-pocket costs is limited.

Q. What is the difference between a nursing home and a skilled nursing facility?

A. This can be very confusing because a nursing home and a skilled nursing facility may be located in the same place or even in the same building. They both may have doctors and nurses on staff.

The difference is that a skilled nursing facility provides medical treatment such as physical rehabilitation services, or medically necessary daily nursing care for the treatment of an illness. A nursing home offers long-term custodial care, which is help with daily activities such as dressing, eating, and bathing.

Q. **What is the difference between an EOMB form and a Notice of Medicare Benefits?**

A. Both are claim notification forms. An EOMB form is used for Part B claims and a Notice of Medicare Benefits is used for Part A claims.

Q. **How is the excess charge calculated?**

A. The excess charge is the difference between the approved charge and the actual charge. For example, if your doctor bills $100 for a service (actual charge) and Medicare allows $80 (approved charge), the excess charge is $20 ($100 − $80 = $20).

Q. **I go to any doctor I want and Medicare pays its portion of the bills. What kind of Medicare coverage do I have?**

A. You are receiving medical care under a fee-for-service type of plan. This is the traditional type of coverage that Medicare has always provided and it is the type of coverage that Medigap policies are designed to supplement.

Q. **If someone in a nursing home is receiving occupational or physical therapy does that mean it is a skilled nursing facility and will be covered by Medicare?**

A. No. A patient in a nursing home who is receiving long-term custodial care may also receive some therapy services, such as speech, physical, or occupational therapy on the premises. These services are offered separately from the routine daily care and may or may not be covered by Medicare, depending upon whether they are deemed medically necessary. These types of therapy sessions would be submitted as Part B expenses.

Q. Are all the Medicare+Choice plans available now?

A. No. Some of the managed care plans currently operating under Medicare (mostly HMOs) will become part of the Medicare+Choice program this year. But there will also be new plans admitted to the program which will expand their availability to Medicare enrollees. The Medical Savings Account (MSA) plans and Private Fee-for-Service Plans, along with the new managed care plans will be available by January 1999.

Q. How do I submit claims for managed care plans?

A. You don't under most circumstances. Generally, you simply pay a co-pay at the time of service and you don't have to do any other paperwork. For plans which allow you to use providers outside the network, you will have to ask the plan administrator how to file the claims as each plan does this differently.

CHAPTER 3

Eligibility for the 65 and Older Crowd

Medicare and Social Security Credits

Medicare was originally targeted to people over age 65 on the assumption that they would be retirees and would be without the benefit of employer-sponsored medical care. The program has never covered people who take early retirement, although there is some discussion now of changing this and including those 62 and older. For 1998, however, the minimum age remains at 65.

Since Medicare was designed as a complement to federal retirement benefits, eligibility is tied closely to eligibility for Social Security benefits. As with Social Security, the availability of coverage is determined by an applicant's age and the length of time s/he (or his/her spouse) has worked in employment qualified under the Social Security Act regulations.

Qualifying Social Security wages are earnings that have had Social Security payroll taxes or Social Security self-employment taxes paid on them. Earnings can qualify if you worked for someone else or for yourself. If you work for someone else, your Social Security payroll taxes are collected and paid by your employer. People who are self-employed pay the Social

Security self-employment tax with their personal income tax return by filing schedule SE.

Whichever work situation applies, the number of Social Security credits needed for Medicare coverage is the same. In 1998, you need to have accumulated 40 quarters of qualified credits to be entitled to Medicare coverage. (For people with fewer quarters of coverage who have attained age 65, there are options which are discussed later.)

When you work in eligible employment, your earnings are tracked throughout your working life, and you receive Social Security earnings credits based on the dollar amount of your earnings each year. Each credit is equal to one calendar quarter of Social Security eligible employment. These credits are accumulated and used to determine your eligibility for Social Security retirement payments and for Medicare coverage. In 1998, a person receives one Social Security credit for each $670 in earnings, up to a maximum of four credits per year. This dollar amount changes as average earning levels of the population rise.

Forty quarters of eligible employment meets the requirement for Medicare eligibility, so if you have accumulated ten years of Social Security eligible earnings you can enroll in Medicare Part A for free and in Part B for the minimum monthly premium.

Because certain types of employment (e.g., federal government workers and nonprofit organization employees) were added to the program fairly recently, it may be possible to qualify for Medicare benefits without having a full 40 quarters of eligible work. Check with Social Security to discuss the specifics of your situation.

Checking for Eligible Work Credits

The accuracy of your employment history is key to obtaining Medicare or Social Security benefits. It is easy to check on the accuracy of your earnings record. The Social Security Administration keeps all records on file based on W-2 employer-reported earnings and Schedule SE self-employment taxes reported. This record is assumed to be accurate, but as with all data it is prudent to check it for yourself periodically. The sooner an error is found, the easier it is to correct and the more likely it is that you will have the necessary documents (such as W-2s) to prove your case.

To check your records, contact the Social Security office and ask for the form entitled Request for Earnings and Benefit Estimate Statement (see following page). After you fill it out and return it to Social Security, you will receive a report listing by year all the eligible employment which Social Security has on file for you. Check this against your records and contact Social Security if there is an error. The report from Social Security will also include an estimate of the Social Security retirement income you will receive.

Special Employment Situations

State and local government workers may or may not be covered, depending upon whether their government employer participates in Social Security. For federal government workers, it depends on their hire date. Generally, federal workers employed after 1983 are eligible for Medicare in the same way private industry workers are because they have paid the Medicare hospital insurance part of the Social Security tax. Federal workers employed before 1983 may qualify to have their work credited toward

Form Approved
OMB No. 0960-0466

SP

Request for Earnings and Benefit Estimate Statement

☐ Please check this box if you want to get your statement in Spanish instead of English.

Please print or type your answers. When you have completed the form, fold it and mail it to us.

1. Name shown on your Social Security card:

First Name _____ Middle Initial ___

Last Name Only

2. Your Social Security number as shown on your card:

☐☐☐ - ☐☐ - ☐☐☐☐

3. Your date of birth

Month | Day | Year

4. Other Social Security numbers you have used:

5. Your sex: ☐ Male ☐ Female

6. Other names you have used
(including a maiden name):
_____

For items 7 and 9 show only earnings covered by Social Security. Do NOT include wages from State, local or Federal Government employment that are NOT covered for Social Security or that are covered ONLY by Medicare.

7. Show your actual earnings (wages and / or net self-employment income) for last year and your estimated earnings for this year.

A. Last year's actual earnings: (*Dollars Only*)

$ ☐☐☐,☐☐☐.00

B. This year's estimated earnings: (*Dollars Only*)

$ ☐☐☐,☐☐☐.00

8. Show the age at which you plan to stop working.
☐☐ (*Show only one age*)

9. Below, show the average yearly amount (not your total future lifetime earnings) that you think you will earn between now and when you plan to stop working. Include cost-of-living, performance or scheduled pay increases or bonuses.

If you expect to earn significantly more or less in the future due to promotions, job changes, part-time work, or an absence from the work force, enter the amount that most closely reflects your future average yearly earnings.

If you don't expect any significant changes, show the same amount you are earning now (the amount in 7B).

Future average yearly earnings: (*Dollars Only*)

$ ☐☐☐,☐☐☐.00

10. Address where you want us to send the statement.

Name _____
Street Address (Include Apt. No., P.O. Box, or Rural Route) _____
City ___ State ___ Zip Code ___

Notice:
I am asking for information about my own Social Security record or the record of a person I am authorized to represent. I understand that when requesting information on a deceased person, I must include proof of death and relationship or appointment. I further understand that if I deliberately request information under false pretenses, I may be guilty of a Federal crime and could be fined and / or imprisoned. I authorize you to use a contractor to send the statement of earnings and benefit estimates to the person named in item 10.

▲

Please sign your name (Do Not Print)

Date ___ (Area Code) Daytime Telephone No. ___

Form **SSA-7004-SM** (4-95) Destroy prior editions   ♻ Printed on recycled paper

Request for Earnings and Benefit Estimate Statement

28

Medicare eligibility under special provisions of the regulations.

State and local government workers became eligible for Medicare qualified employment in 1986. Whether or not work prior to 1986 will qualify depends on their government's agreement with Social Security.

There are special regulations covering people who were employed in domestic work, farm work, or religious organizations that were exempt from Social Security tax payments. All of these atypical situations must be evaluated on a case by case basis. This is best done by speaking with a Social Security representative.

Other Eligibility Requirements

In addition to the number of work credits accumulated, there are other requirements for Medicare enrollment. To be eligible for Medicare, an applicant must be 65 years of age or older and be either:

- a United States citizen (by birth or naturalization), or

- a legal resident alien who has lived in the United States for at least five years.

If you are over 65 and any of the following applies to you, you are eligible for Medicare benefits:

- You currently receive Social Security or Railroad Retirement Board benefits.

- You are qualified to receive Social Security or Railroad Retirement Board benefits because you have worked long enough to be eligible, even though you have not applied for them.

- Your spouse (or divorced spouse) is at least 62 years of age and is eligible based on his/her work record.

- You worked long enough in an eligible federal, state, or local government job to be eligible under the Social Security Act regulations.

Eligibility Based on the Work History of Others

Once they have reached age 65, divorced spouses, widows and widowers, and dependent parents can be eligible for benefits based on a spouse or child's work record. If you are using your child's employment history, you must prove that the child contributes at least one-half of your support.

Generally, you must have been married for ten years to use your spouse or ex-spouse's work record for eligibility or married for at least one year to use your deceased spouse's work record. Your local Social Security office can check on the applicability of any of these options for you.

How to Enroll in Medicare

If you are already receiving Social Security benefits or Railroad Retirement Board benefits at the time you turn 65 (perhaps you elected to take retirement at an earlier age), you will be enrolled automatically. Otherwise, you must apply to receive benefits.

A few months before your 65th birthday, you should receive a notice explaining how to sign up. Enrollment in Medicare should be done approximately three months before your 65th birthday, in order to make certain that you receive your benefits as soon as you turn 65.

It is not necessary for you to retire in order to receive Medicare coverage; you simply must meet the requirements outlined earlier. By enrolling three months in advance of your 65th birthday, you will avoid possible delays in your coverage and will ensure that you do not miss your initial enrollment opportunity.

Timely enrollment is important because there are restrictions on when you may enroll in Medicare Part B. Your enrollment date affects when your benefits begin and how much they cost.

Make an appointment at your local Social Security office to complete an application. Most of the information will be entered directly into the computer by the Social Security office employee. The application form is reproduced here (see next page) to show the questions that you will be asked. (If you have already filed for Social Security retirement benefits, you should also have filed for Medicare benefits. If so, you do not need to file another form.)

To make the application process as quick and smooth as possible, bring the following information with you to your appointment:

- Your Social Security card, or the number if you have lost your card.

- Your tax returns or w-2 forms for the last two years. The records in the Social Security data center are often behind by one or two years. Bringing this information will provide proof of your eligible wages and aid in calculating your eligibility.

- Proof of your age, preferably a birth certificate.

DEPARTMENT OF HEALTH AND HUMAN SERVICES
HEALTH CARE FINANCING ADMINISTRATION

Form Approved
OMB NO. 0938-0251

(Do Not Write in this space)

APPLICATION FOR HOSPITAL INSURANCE

(This application form may also be used to
enroll in Supplementary Medical Insurance)

I apply for entitlement to Medicare's hospital insurance under part A of title XVIII of the Social Security Act, as presently amended, and for any cash benefits to which I may be entitled under title II of that Act.

1.	(a) Print your name ⟶	(First name, middle initial, last name)
	(b) Enter your name at birth if different from 1 (a) ⟶	
	(c) Enter your sex (check one) ⟶	☐ Male ☐ Female
2.	Enter your Social Security Number ⟶	_ _ _/_ _/_ _ _ _
3.	(a) Enter your date of birth (Month, day, year) ⟶	
	(b) Enter name of State or foreign country where you were born ⟶	
	If you have already submitted a public or religious record of your birth made before you were age 5, go on to item 4)	
	(c) Was a public record of your birth made before you were age 5?	☐ Yes ☐ No ☐ Unknown
	(d) Was a religious record of your birth made before you were age 5?	☐ Yes ☐ No ☐ Unknown
4.	(a) Have you (or has someone on your behalf) ever filed an application for social security benefits, a period of disability under social security, supplemental security income, or hospital or medical insurance under Medicare? ⟶	☐ Yes ☐ No
(If "Yes" answer (b) and (c).)   *(If "No," go on to item 5.)*
	(b) Enter name of person on whose social security record you filed other application ⟶	
	(c) Enter Social Security Number of person named in (b), *(If unknown, so indicate)* ⟶	_ _ _/_ _/_ _ _ _
5.	(a) Were you in the active military or naval service (including Reserve or National Guard *active* duty or active duty for training) after September 7, 1939? ⟶	☐ Yes ☐ No
(If "Yes" answer (b) and (c).)   *(If "No," go on to item 6.)*
	(b) Enter dates of service ⟶	*From: (Month, year) To: (Month, year)*
	(c) Have you *ever* been (or will you be) eligible for a monthly benefit from a military or civilian Federal agency? (Include Veterans Administration benefits *only* if you waived military retirement pay) ⟶	☐ Yes ☐ No
6.	Did you work in the railroad industry any time on or after January 1, 1937? ⟶	☐ Yes ☐ No

Form HCFA-18 F5 (10-84) Page 1   (Over)

Application for Enrollment,
Page 1

7.	(a) Have you ever engaged in work that was covered under the social security system of a country other than the United States? ⟶		☐ Yes	☐ No		
	(b) If "Yes," list the country(ies). ⟶					
8.	(a) How much were your total earnings last year? ⟶ *(If none, write "None")*	Earnings $				
	(b) How much do you expect your total earnings to be this year? ⟶ *(If none, write "None")*	Earnings $				
9.	Are you a resident of the United States? ⟶ *(To reside in a place means to make a home there.)*		☐ Yes	☐ No		
10.	(a) Are you a citizen of the United States? ⟶ *(If "Yes," go on to item 11.)(If "No," answer (b) and (c) below.)*		☐ Yes	☐ No		
	(b) Are you lawfully admitted for permanent residence in the United States? ⟶		☐ Yes	☐ No		

(c) Enter below the information requested about your place of residence in the last 5 years:

ADDRESS AT WHICH YOU RESIDED IN THE LAST 5 YEARS (Begin with the most recent address. Show actual date residence began even if that is prior to the last 5 years.)	DATE RESIDENCE BEGAN			DATE RESIDENCE ENDED		
	Month	Day	Year	Month	Day	Year

(If you need more space, use the "Remarks" space on the third page or another sheet of paper)

11.	Are you currently married? ⟶		☐ Yes	☐ No
YOUR CURRENT MARRIAGE	*(If "Yes," give the following information about your current marriage.) (If "No," go on to item 12.)*			
	To whom married (Enter your wife's maiden name or your husband's name.)	When (Month, day, year)		
	Spouse's date of birth (or age)	Spouse's Social Security Number *(If none or unknown, so indicate)* __ __ __ / __ __ / __ __ __ __		

12.	If you had a previous marriage and your spouse died, OR if you had a previous marriage which lasted 10 or more years, give the following information. *(If you had no previous marriage(s), enter "NONE.")*	
YOUR PREVIOUS MARRIAGE	To whom married *(Enter your wife's maiden name or your husband's name.)*	When (Month, day, year)
	Spouse's date of birth (or age)	Spouse's Social Security Number *(If none or unknown, so indicate)* __ __ __ / __ __ / __ __ __ __
	If spouse deceased, give date of death ⟶	

(Use "Remarks" space on page 3 for information about any other marriages.)

Form HCFA-18 F5 (10-84) Page 2

Application for Enrollment,
Page 2

13.	Is or was your spouse a railroad worker, railroad retirement pensioner, or a railroad retirement annuitant?	☐ Yes	☐ No
14.	(a)Were you or your spouse a civilian employee of the Federal Government after June 1960? *(If "Yes," answer (b).) (If "No," omit (b), (c), and (d).)*	☐ Yes	☐ No
	(b)Are you or your spouse now covered under a medical insurance plan provided by the Federal Employees Health Benefits Act of 1959? *(If "Yes," omit (c) and (d).) (If "No," answer (c).)*	☐ Yes	☐ No
	(c)Are you **and** your spouse barred from coverage under the above Act because your Federal employment, or your spouse's was not long enough? *(If "Yes," omit (d) and explain in "Remarks" below.) (If "No," answer (d).)*	☐ Yes	☐ No
	(d)Were either you or your spouse an employee of the Federal Government after February 15, 1965?	☐ Yes	☐ No

Remarks:

15.	If you are found to be otherwise ineligible for hospital insurance under Medicare, do you wish to enroll for hospital insurance on a monthly premium basis (in addition to the monthly premium for supplementary medical insurance)? *(If "Yes," you MUST also sign up for medical insurance.)*	☐ Yes	☐ No

INFORMATION ON MEDICAL INSURANCE UNDER MEDICARE

Medical insurance under Medicare helps pay your doctor bills. It also helps pay for a number of other medical items and services not covered under the hospital insurance part of Medicare.

If you sign up for medical insurance, you must pay a premium for each month you have this protection. If you get monthly social security, railroad retirement, or civil service benefits, your premium will be deducted from your benefit check, if you get none of these benefits, you will be notified how to pay your premium.

The Federal Government contributes to the cost of your insurance. The amount of your premium and the Government's payment are based on the cost of services covered by medical insurance. The Government also makes additional payments when necessary to meet the full cost of the program. (Currently, the Government pays about two-thirds of the cost of this program.) You will get advance notice if there is any change in your premium amount.

If you have questions or would like a leaflet on medical insurance, call any Social Security office.

SEE OTHER SIDE TO SIGN UP FOR MEDICAL INSURANCE

Form HCFA-18 F5 (10-84) Page 3   (Over)

Application for Enrollment, Page 3

If you become entitled to hospital insurance as a result of this application, you will be enrolled for medical insurance automatically unless you indicate below that you do not want this protection. If you decline to enroll now, you can get medical insurance protection later only if you sign up for it during specified enrollment periods. Your protection may then be delayed and you may have to pay a higher premium when you decide to sign up.

The date your medical insurance begins and the amount of the premium you must pay depend on the month you file this application with the Social Security Administration. Any social security office will be glad to explain the rules regarding enrollment to you.

16.	**DO YOU WISH TO ENROLL FOR SUPPLEMENTARY MEDICAL INSURANCE?** ➤	☐ Yes ☐ No
	(If "Yes," answer question 17.)	
	(Enrollees for premium hospital insurance must simultaneously enroll for medical insurance.)	☐ Currently Enrolled
17.	Are you or your spouse receiving an annuity under the Federal Civil Service Retirement Act or other law administered by the Office of Personnel Management? ➤	☐ Yes ☐ No
	(If "Yes," enter Civil Service annuity number here. Include the prefix	Your No.
	"CSA" for annuitant, "CSF" for survivor.)	Spouse's No.
	If you entered your spouse's number, is he (she) enrolled for supplementary medical insurance under social security? ➤	☐ Yes ☐ No

I know that anyone who makes or causes to be made a false statement or representation of material fact in a application or for use in determining a right to payment under the Social Security Act commits a crime punishable under Federal law by fine, imprisonment or both. I affirm that all information I have given in this document is true.

SIGNATURE OF APPLICANT	Date *(Month, day year)*
Signature *(First name, middle initial, last name) (Write in Ink)* **SIGN HERE** ➤	Telephone Number(s) at which you may be contacted during the day

Mailing address *(Number and street, Apt. No., P.O. Box, or Rural Route)*

City and State	ZIP Code	Enter Name of County (if any) in which you now live

Witnesses are required ONLY if this application has been signed by mark (X) above. If signed by mark (X), two witnesses to the signing who know the applicant must sign below, giving their full addresses.

1. Signature of Witness	2. Signature of Witness
Address *(Number and street, City, State, and ZIP Code)*	Address *(Number and street, City, State, and ZIP Code)*

Form HCFA-18 F5 (10-84) Page 4   ☆U.S. Government Printing Office: 1986-607-648

Application for Enrollment,
Page 4

A REMINDER TO APPLICANTS FOR THE SOCIAL SECURITY HOSPITAL INSURANCE

NAME OF PERSON TO CONTACT ABOUT YOUR CLAIM	SSA OFFICE	DATE
TELEPHONE NO.		

RECEIPT FOR YOU CLAIM

Your application for the hospital insurance has been received and will be processed as quickly as possible.

You should hear from us within _____ days after you have given us all the information we requested. Some claims may take longer if additional information is needed.

In the meantime, if you change your mailing address, you should report the change.

Always give us your claim number when writing or telephoning about your claim.

If you have any questions about your claim, we will be glad to help you.

CLAIMANT	SOCIAL SECURITY CLAIM NUMBER

COLLECTION AND USE OF INFORMATION FROM YOUR APPLICATION — PRIVACY ACT NOTICE

PRIVACY ACT NOTICE: The Social Security Administration (SSA) is authorized to collect the information on this form under sections 226 and 1818 of the Social Security Act, as amended (42 U.S.C. 426 and 1395-17) and section 103 of Public Law 89-97. The information on this form is needed to enable social security and the Health Care Financing Administration (HCFA) to determine if you and your dependents may be entitled to hospital and/or medical insurance coverage and/or monthly benefits. While you do not have to furnish the information requested on this form to social security, no benefits or hospital or medical insurance can be provided until an application has been received by a social security office. Failure to provide all or part of the information requested could prevent an accurate and timely decision on your claim or your dependent's claim, and could result in the loss of some benefits of hospital or medical insurance. Although the information you furnish on this form is almost never used for any other purpose than stated above, there is a possibility that for the administration of social security or HCFA programs or for the administration of programs requiring coordination with SSA or HCFA, information may be disclosed to another person or to another governmental agency as follows: 1) to enable a third party or an agency to assist social security or HCFA in establishing rights to social security benefits and/or hospital or medical insurance coverage; 2) to comply with Federal laws requiring the release of information from social security and HCFA records (e.g., to the General Accounting Office and the Veterans Administration); and 3) to facilitate statistical research and audit activities necessary to assure the integrity and improvement of the social security and HCFA programs (e.g., to the Bureau of the Census and private concerns under contract to social security and HCFA).

Form HCFA-18 F5 (10-84) Page 5

**Application for Enrollment,
Page 5**

Other types of proof are acceptable, such as naturalization certificates, passports, hospital birth records, military records, or other records that establish your age.

- Military service record. Active duty military service can increase your number of credits.

- Evidence of legal name changes, if any.

If you are applying based on another person's employment record, bring any of the following documentation that applies:

- Your spouse's, ex-spouse's, or late spouse's Social Security number or card

- Your marriage certificate, spouse's death certificate, or divorce decree

- Your child's Social Security card or number if you are filing as a dependent parent

- Proof that your child is responsible for half or more of your annual support

Part B Enrollment Periods

Part B coverage is controlled by enrollment periods. You must apply during an enrollment period and the effective date of your coverage may be delayed if you do not file in a timely manner.

The initial enrollment period for Part B coverage is seven months long. It begins three months before your 65th birthday and ends three months after the month in which you are 65, for a total of seven months including the month of your birthday.

Initial Enrollment Periods

Birthday month	Beginning of Application Period	End of Application Period
January	October	April
February	November	May
March	December	June
April	January	July
May	February	August
June	March	September
July	April	October
August	May	November
September	June	December
October	July	January
November	August	February
December	September	March

If you miss your initial enrollment period or decline Part B coverage when you apply for Medicare Part A, you must wait until the next general Medicare Part B enrollment period to apply. This open enrollment opportunity begins January 1 and runs until March 31 each year. Coverage applied for during this time begins on the following July 1. If you delay applying for more than 12 months after the initial enrollment period, your monthly premium charges for coverage may be higher, amounting to an extra ten percent for each 12 month period you have delayed.

If the delay in enrollment is because you were covered by your own or your spouse's employer sponsored group health care plan, the extra charge may not apply. You are eligible to enroll without the ten percent annual premium increase if you enroll within the eight-month period after your participation in the employer's plan is ended.

Denial of Application

If your application is denied, the first step is to find out why you were turned down. Question the explanation for denial until you are certain that you understand what the problem is.

If the denial is due to lack of information or incorrect information, the situation is relatively easy to remedy. For instance, errors involving your earnings record, residency requirements, or date of birth can usually be corrected by contacting your local Social Security office and providing them with the necessary proof. If you have too few quarters of work credit, you may be able to earn them by working in eligible employment now. Or, you may be able to use a spouse's work record to qualify. Don't hesitate to explore all options with the Social Security office.

People Not Eligible for Medicare

If you do not qualify for Medicare Part A or Part B under the rules discussed earlier, it may still be possible for you to get Medicare coverage — it will be more expensive for you than for qualified Medicare recipients, however.

If you are age 65 or older and a United States citizen, but do not meet the Medicare work credit requirements, you may be able to purchase both Part A and Part B insurance for a monthly fee. If you are a resident alien, you may also purchase coverage, but you must have resided in the United States for five years in order to purchase Medicare Part B coverage.

If you wish to enroll in Medicare, you are eligible to do so during the January 1 to March 31 open enrollment period each year. If you are not eligible for free coverage under Part A, you must enroll in both Part A and Part B to obtain Part A coverage. Part B coverage can be purchased without Part A, but Part A cannot be purchased by itself.

To apply, you will need to make an appointment at your Social Security office and complete the application shown on pages 32–36. Although the application title refers to hospital insurance, the form includes a section where you can enroll in Part B as well.

Frequently Asked Questions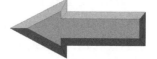

Q. Who is eligible for Medicare?

A. U.S. citizens and legal resident aliens age 65 and over can qualify for premium-free Part A benefits if they can establish their eligibility based on their own, their spouse's, ex-spouse's or late spouse's work record. Government employees who worked in Medicare-eligible employment, and their spouses, can also qualify.

Coverage is also available to most individuals suffering from permanent kidney failure, and to those who have been entitled to Social Security disability benefits or Railroad Retirement disability benefits for more than 24 months, and to certain disabled government employees whose work has been covered for Medicare purposes.

Anyone who is eligible for Part A is eligible for Part B benefits as well. There is a monthly premium for Part B benefits.

Q. I have Part A, but not Part B. How much will it cost and how do I enroll?

A. The base cost in 1998 for Part B for eligible beneficiaries is $43.80 per month. Call your local Social Security office (listed in the phone book under United States Government) or the national office (800-772-1213, TTY 800-325-0778), and they can give you information about the costs involved in your particular situation.

If your initial enrollment period has ended, you may enroll during the yearly general enrollment period of January 1 through March 31. Your coverage will be effective on July 1 of that year.

Q. I signed up for Part B coverage a couple of years after I enrolled in Part A. Why is my monthly premium more than $43.80?

A. If you don't sign up for Part B coverage when you first become eligible, Medicare charges you a slightly higher premium based on the number of years in which you did not have coverage. The premium is increased by 10 percent for each year you weren't enrolled. There are exceptions to this policy, so be sure to tell the Medicare representative why you did not enroll earlier in case you qualify for the lower premium.

Q. How do I sign up for Medicare?

A. If you are receiving Social Security or Railroad Retirement benefit payments when you turn 65, you should automatically get a Medicare card in the mail. If you apply for Social Security retirement benefits, you will apply for Medicare at the same time.

If you are not receiving such payments, or you do not

intend to apply for retirement benefits, you will have to apply for Medicare coverage. Call Social Security to make an appointment and bring all the items previously listed in this chapter with you.

Once enrolled, you will be issued a card that will show whether you are enrolled in both Part A and Part B along with the beginning dates of coverage for each.

Q. **I need to file for Medicare. When should I do it?**

A. File the application for Medicare during the initial seven-month enrollment period that starts three months before the month you turn 65. If this period is over, you may apply during the January 1 to March 31 general enrollment period in any year.

Q. **I have Part B coverage, but I don't want it. What do I do?**

A. If you do not want Part B you can refuse it by following the instructions that came with the card when you first enrolled. If you have been enrolled for awhile, call or visit your Social Security office and ask them to remove the coverage.

Q. **When I enrolled in Medicare Part A, I did not sign up for Part B. Can I still get coverage?**

A. You can enroll in Part B during the general enrollment period from January 1 to March 31 each year. Your coverage won't begin until July 1 of the year you enroll. Because you delayed enrollment your monthly premium may be higher than it would have been had you enrolled in Part B when you enrolled in Part A. The usual surcharge is ten percent for each 12 month period in which you could have been enrolled but were not. This surcharge is waived in some circumstances, so you should check with Social Security for the exact cost to you.

Q. I did not enroll in Medicare because I was covered under my employer's group health plan. As I am no longer covered under this plan, how do I get Medicare?

A. There is a special enrollment period that applies in this situation. You may enroll in Medicare during the eight-month period following the termination of your group health benefits.

Q. I am 63, retired, and receiving Social Security retirement benefits. Can I get Medicare coverage?

A. No. Not until you are 65, at which time you should be automatically enrolled in both Part A and Part B.

Q. I am not eligible for Medicare based on my employment history. Is there any way to get coverage?

A. Yes. If you are age 65 or over and a United States citizen (or a resident alien who has been lawfully admitted for permanent residence and has resided in the United States for at least five years), you can obtain either or both types of Medicare coverage (Part A and/or Part B) by paying a monthly premium. You will have to pay a premium for both Part A coverage and Part B coverage. Depending upon the number of credits you need, you could work additional time in Social Security eligible employment to earn the needed credits.

Q. My employment record at Social Security is wrong. What should I do?

A. Put together documentation of your correct wage history and call Social Security to get instructions for correcting the error. You may be able to correct the information on the phone, or you may have to go to your local Social Security office and meet with a representative. It depends upon the type of error that needs to be corrected.

Q. How often should I check my earnings record?

A. It is prudent to check it every three years until you apply for benefits. This allows mistakes to be corrected early.

Q. I don't have 40 quarters of credits, but I was in the military service. Does that have any effect on my eligibility?

A. Yes. Basic pay earned during active duty military service or active duty for training earns credits. If the service was after 1957, the credits should show on your earnings statement. If you served between 1940 and 1957, contact your Social Security office to find out how many credits you earned based on your military service.

Q. I am a widow without 40 credits of qualifying employment. Can I apply based on my husband's work history?

A. Yes. Bring your late husband's Social Security number, your marriage certificate, and his death certificate with you when you apply for Medicare benefits.

Q. I have been turned down for Medicare coverage because the records do not show all my earnings. What can I do?

A. Contact your local Social Security office and bring copies of your tax returns, w-2 forms, and any other documentation you have to prove your employment history. Also bring proof of any active duty military service, as this can help contribute to the total number of needed quarters.

Q. Most of my employment was as a domestic worker. Am I eligible for Medicare?

A. Check with Social Security to find out how you can qualify. There are special rules that apply to domestic workers and farm workers.

Q. I don't have 40 quarters of eligible employment. How much will it cost for me to purchase Part A insurance?

A. In 1998, if you have between 30 and 40 quarters of credits, it costs $170 per month. If you have fewer than 30 quarters of credit, it is $309 per month.

Q. I worked for a non-profit organization. Will my employment qualify me for Medicare?

A. There are special rules which apply. Check with Social Security for specifics on your situation.

Q. Will my military service count toward my Social Security credits?

A. Yes, if it was active duty service. Service before 1957 may not show up on your Social Security earnings record, so make sure that Social Security has all the details about your length and type of service.

CHAPTER 4

Medicare and
the Disabled

**Medicare
Coverage**

Medicare is primarily thought of as a benefit for the elderly, but benefits are available for the disabled, including people being treated for kidney failure. Medicare eligibility based on disability is available without regard to age provided the applicant is a United States citizen or permanent legal resident. Currently, approximately four million people receive Medicare benefits due to disability or treatment for kidney failure.

The requirements for eligibility are different from those for the elderly. If you are already eligible for, or are receiving Medicare benefits as a person over age 65, you will not be eligible for separate disability benefits. Your coverage will be under the regular Medicare provisions for those over 65.

**Disability
Eligibility**

Medicare's definition of disability is quite stringent and differs from the standards set by other agencies or private insurers. You must prove that you are unable to hold gainful employment in any job in order to meet Medicare's definition of permanently and totally disabled. Medicare's definition mirrors the requirements of Social

Security's definition of disability. In addition, you must be either a United States citizen (by birth or naturalization) or a resident alien who has resided in the United States for at least five years.

If you meet any one of the following conditions, you will qualify for Medicare under the disability provisions:

- You have received Social Security disability benefits for 24 months or more.

- You have worked long enough in a federal, state, or local government job to qualify, and you meet the requirements of the Social Security disability program.

- You receive disability benefits from the Railroad Retirement Board and have fulfilled a Medicare waiting period requirement.

There is a five-month waiting period before you receive Medicare benefits. The waiting period begins with the date you qualify for benefits, not the day you apply for them.

Applying for Medicare Disability Benefits

If you have received disability benefits under the Social Security or Railroad Retirement Board programs for 24 months, you will receive notification automatically about your eligibility for Medicare. If you are not a beneficiary of either of these programs, you will have to apply for Medicare benefits.

To apply, you will need evidence of the nature and extent of your disability. You will also need to satisfy the requirement for certain minimum numbers of eligible Social Security

---

DEPARTMENT OF HEALTH AND HUMAN SERVICES
Social Security Administration   ☐ TEL   Form Approved
OMB No. 0960-0060   TOE 120/145

(Do not write in this space)

APPLICATION FOR DISABILITY INSURANCE BENEFITS

I apply for a period of disability and/or all insurance benefits for which I am eligible under title II and part A of title XVIII of the Social Security Act, as presently amended.

PART I—INFORMATION ABOUT THE DISABLED WORKER

1. (a) PRINT your name   ⟶   FIRST NAME, MIDDLE INITIAL, LAST NAME

     (b) Enter your name at birth if different from item (a)   ⟶

     (c) Check (✓) whether you are   ⟶   ☐ Male   ☐ Female

2. Enter your Social Security Number   ⟶   _ _ _ / _ _ / _ _ _ _

3. (a) Enter your date of birth   ⟶   MONTH, DAY, YEAR

     (b) Enter name of State or foreign country where you were born   ⟶

If you have already presented, or if you are now presenting, a public or religious record of your birth established before you were age 5, go on to item 4.

     (c) Was a public record of your birth made before you were age 5?   ☐ Yes   ☐ No   ☐ Unknown

     (d) Was a religious record of your birth made before you were age 5?   ☐ Yes   ☐ No   ☐ Unknown

4. (a) What is your disabling condition? (Briefly describe the injury or illness that prevents, or has prevented, you from working.)

     (b) Is your injury or illness related to your work in any way?   ⟶   ☐ Yes   ☐ No

5. (a) When did you become unable to work because of your disabling condition?   MONTH, DAY, YEAR

     (b) Are you still disabled? (If "Yes," go on to item 6.) If "No," answer (c).)   ☐ Yes   ☐ No

     (c) If you are no longer disabled, enter the date your disability ended.   ⟶   MONTH, DAY, YEAR

6. (a) Have you (or has someone on your behalf) ever filed an application for Social Security benefits, a period of disability under Social Security, supplemental security income, or hospital or medical insurance under Medicare?   ⟶   ☐ Yes   ☐ No   ☐ Unknown
(If "Yes," answer (b) and (c).)   (If "No," or "Unknown" go on to item 7.)

     (b) Enter name of person on whose Social Security record you filed other application.

     (c) Enter Social Security Number of person named in (b). If unknown, check this block. ☐   ⟶   _ _ _ / _ _ / _ _ _ _

7. (a) Were you in the active military or naval service (including Reserve or National Guard active duty or active duty for training) after September 7, 1939 and before 1968?   ☐ Yes   ☐ No
(If "Yes," answer (b) and (c).)   (If "No," go on to item 8.)

     (b) Enter dates of service   ⟶   FROM: (month, year)   TO:(month, year)

     (c) Have you _ever_ been (or will you be) eligible for a monthly benefit from a military or civilian Federal agency? (include Veterans Administration benefits _only_ if you waived military retirement pay)   ⟶   ☐ Yes   ☐ No

Form **SSA-16-F6** (7-93)   Page 1   ♻ Printed on recycled paper

Application for Disability Insurance Benefits, Page 1

8.	(a) Have you filed (or do you intend to file) for any other public disability benefits? (Include workers' compensation and Black Lung benefits)	☐ Yes (If "Yes," answer (b).)	☐ No (If "No," go on to item 9.)

(b) The other public disability benefit(s) you have filed (or intend to file) for is (Check as many as apply):
- ☐ Veterans Administration Benefits
- ☐ Supplemental Security Income
- ☐ Welfare
- ☐ Other (If "Other," complete a Workers' Compensation/Public Disability Benefit Questionnaire)

9.	(a) Do you have social security credits (for example, based on work or residence) under another country's Social Security System? (If "Yes," answer (b).) (If "No," go on to item 10.)	☐ Yes	☐ No

(b) List the country(ies):

10.	(a) Are you entitled to, or do you expect to become entitled to, a pension or annuity based on your work after 1956 not covered by Social Security?	☐ Yes (If "Yes," answer (b) and (c).)	☐ No (If "No," go on to item 11.)

(b) ☐ I became entitled, or expect to become entitled, beginning — MONTH / YEAR

(c) ☐ I became eligible, or expect to become eligible, beginning — MONTH / YEAR

I agree to notify the Social Security Administration if I become entitled to a pension or annuity based on my employment after 1956 not covered by Social Security, or if such pension or annuity stops.

11.	(a) Did you have wages or self-employment income covered under Social Security in all years from 1978 through last year?	☐ Yes (If "Yes," skip to item 12.)	☐ No (If "No," answer (b).)

(b) List the years from 1978 through last year in which you did not have wages or self-employment income covered under Social Security.

12. Enter below the names and addresses of all the persons, companies, or Government agencies for whom you have worked this year and last year. IF NONE, WRITE "NONE" BELOW AND GO ON TO ITEM 14.

NAME AND ADDRESS OF EMPLOYER (If you had more than one employer, please list them in order beginning with your last (most recent) employer)	Work Began MONTH	YEAR	Work Ended (If still working show "Not ended") MONTH	YEAR

(If you need more space, use "Remarks" space on page 4.)

13.	May the Social Security Administration or the State agency reviewing your case ask your employers for information needed to process your claim?	☐ Yes	☐ No

14. **THIS ITEM MUST BE COMPLETED, EVEN IF YOU WERE AN EMPLOYEE.**

(a) Were you self-employed this year and last year? (If "Yes," answer (b).) (If "No," go on to item 15.)	☐ Yes	☐ No

(b) Check the year or years in which you were self-employed	In what kind of trade or business were you self-employed? (For example, storekeeper, farmer, physician)	Were your net earnings from your trade or business $400 or more? (Check "Yes" or "No")	
☐ This Year			
☐ Last Year		☐ Yes	☐ No
☐ Year before last		☐ Yes	☐ No

15.	(a) How much were your total earnings last year? (Count both wages and self-employment income. If none, write "None.")	Amount $_____
	(b) How much have you earned so far this year? (If none, write "None.")	Amount $_____

Form **SSA-16-F6** (7-93)　　　Page 2

Application for Disability Insurance Benefits, Page 2

(c) Did you receive any money from an employer(s) on or after the date in item 5(a) when you became unable to work because of your disability? (If "Yes," give amounts and explain in "Remarks" on page 4.) →		☐ Yes Amount $_____	☐ No
(d) Do you expect to receive any additional money from an employer such as sick pay, vacation pay, other special pay? (If "Yes," please give amounts and explain in "Remarks" on page 4.) →		☐ Yes Amount $_____	☐ No

PART II—INFORMATION ABOUT THE DISABLED WORKER AND SPOUSE

16.	Have you ever been married? → (If "Yes," answer item 17.) (If "No," go on to item 18.)	☐ Yes	☐ No

17. (a) Give the following information about your current marriage. If not currently married, show your last marriage below.

To whom married		When (Month, day, year)	Where (Name of City and State)
Your current or last marriage	How marriage ended (If still in effect, write "Not ended.")	When (Month, day, year)	Where (Name of City and State)
	Marriage performed by ☐ Clergyman or public official ☐ Other (Explain in Remarks)	Spouse's date of birth (or age)	If spouse deceased, give date of death
	Spouse's Social Security Number (If none or unknown, so indicate)		__ __ __ / __ __ / __ __ __ __

(b) Give the following information about each of your previous marriages. (**If none, write "NONE."**)

To whom married		When (Month, day, year)	Where (Name of City and State)
Your previous marriage	How marriage ended	When (Month, day, year)	Where (Name of City and State)
	Marriage performed by ☐ Clergyman or public official ☐ Other (Explain in Remarks)	Spouse's date of birth (or age)	If spouse is deceased, give date of death
	Spouse's Social Security Number (If none or unknown, so indicate)		__ __ __ / __ __ / __ __ __ __

(Use a separate statement for information about any other marriages.)

18.	Have you or your spouse worked in the railroad industry for 7 years or more? →	☐ Yes	☐ No

PART III—INFORMATION ABOUT THE DEPENDENTS OF THE DISABLED WORKER

19. If your claim for disability benefits is approved, your children (including natural children, adopted children, and stepchildren) or dependent grandchildren (including stepgrandchildren) may be eligible for benefits based on your earnings record.

List below: FULL NAME OF ALL such children who are now or were in the past 12 months UNMARRIED and:
- UNDER AGE 18
- AGE 18 TO 19 AND ATTENDING SECONDARY SCHOOL
- DISABLED OR HANDICAPPED (age 18 or over and disability began before age 22)
- **(IF THERE ARE NO SUCH CHILDREN, WRITE "NONE" BELOW AND GO ON TO ITEM 20.)**

20.	Do you have a dependent parent who was receiving at least one-half support from you when you became unable to work because of your disability? (If "Yes," enter name and address in "Remarks" on page 4.)	☐ Yes	☐ No

Form **SSA-16-F6** (7-93)   Page 3

Application for Disability Insurance Benefits, Page 3

**IMPORTANT INFORMATION ABOUT DISABILITY INSURANCE BENEFITS—
PLEASE READ CAREFULLY**

I. **SUBMITTING MEDICAL EVIDENCE:** I understand that as a claimant for disability benefits, I am responsible for providing medical evidence showing the nature and extent of my disability. I may be asked either to submit the evidence myself or to assist the Social Security Administration in obtaining the evidence. If such evidence is not sufficient to arrive at a determination, I may be requested by the State Disability Determination Service to have an independent examination at the expense of the Social Security Administration.

II. **RELEASE OF INFORMATION:** I authorize any physician, hospital, agency or other organization to disclose to the Social Security Administration, or to the State Agency that may review my claim or continuing disability, any medical record or other information about my disability.

I also authorize the Social Security Administration to release medical information from my records, only as necessary to process my claim, as follows:
- Copies of medical information may be provided to a physician or medical institution prior to my appearance for an independent medical examination if an examination is necessary.
- Results of any such independent examination may be provided to my personal physician.
- Information may be furnished to any contractor for transcription, typing, record copying, or other related clerical or administrative service performed for the State Disability Determination Service.
- The State Vocational Rehabilitation Agency may review any evidence necessary for determining my eligibility for rehabilitative services.

THIS MUST BE ANSWERED ▶ **21. DO YOU UNDERSTAND AND AGREE WITH THE AUTHORIZATIONS GIVE ABOVE?**

☐ Yes   ☐ No   (If "No," explain why in "Remarks.")

22. Check if applicable:
( ) I am not submitting evidence of ( ) my ( ) the deceased's earnings that are not yet on ( ) my ( ) his/her earnings record. I understand that these earnings will be included automatically within 24 months, and any increase in benefits will be paid with full retroactivity.

REMARKS (You may use this space for any explanation. If you need more space, attach a separate sheet.)

III. **REPORTING RESPONSIBILITIES:** I agree to promptly notify Social Security if:
- My MEDICAL CONDITION IMPROVES so that I would be able to work, even though I have not yet returned to work.
- I GO TO WORK whether as an employee or a self-employed person.
- I apply for or begin to receive a worker's compensation (including black lung benefits) or another public disability benefit, or the amount that I am receiving changes or stops, or I receive a lump-sum settlement.
- I am imprisoned for conviction of a felony.

The above events may affect my eligibility to disability benefits as provided in the Social Security Act, as amended.

I know that anyone who makes or causes to be made a false statement or representation of material fact in an application or for use in determining a right to payment under the Social Security Act commits a crime punishable under Federal law by fine, imprisonment or both. I affirm that all information I have given in this document is true.

SIGNATURE OF APPLICANT | DATE (Month, day, year)

SIGNATURE (First name, middle initial, last name) (Write in ink.)

SIGN HERE ▶ | Telephone Number(s) at which you may be contacted during the day. (Include the area code)

	Direct Deposit Payment Address *(Financial Institution)*				
FOR OFFICIAL USE ONLY	Routing Transit Number	C/S	Depositor Account Number	☐ No Account	
				☐ Direct Deposit Refused	

Applicant's Mailing Address *(Number and street, Apt. No., P.O. Box, or Rural Route)* *(Enter Residence Address in "Remarks," if different.)*

City and State	ZIP Code	County *(if any)* in which you now live

Witnesses are required ONLY if this application has been signed by mark (X) above. If signed by mark (X), two witnesses to the signing who know the applicant must sign below, giving their full addresses. Also, print the applicant's name in Signature block.

1. Signature of Witness	2. Signature of Witness
Address *(Number and street, City, State and ZIP Code)*	Address *(Number and street, City, State and ZIP Code)*

Form **SSA-16-F6** (7-93)   Page 4

Application for Disability Insurance Benefits, Page 4

employment quarters. The total number of employment quarters required to receive Medicare disability benefits varies according to the age at which you became totally disabled. These work credits are calculated in the same manner as was discussed in the previous chapter. Generally:

■ If you are 18 to 23 you will need credit for six quarters of eligible work in the three years before your disability began.

■ If you are 24 to 30 you will need a sufficient number of quarters to equal one-half the number of quarters possible between the age of 21 and the age at which you became disabled.

■ If you are 31 or older you will need between 20 and 40 quarters of work credit, depending upon the age at which you became disabled and your date of birth. At least 20 of the credits must have been earned in the 10 years immediately prior to your becoming disabled. The chart below outlines the credits needed in this situation.

In the event you are able to return to work, it may be possible to extend your Medicare benefit coverage for up to 24 months. In all instances, eligibility for benefits should be discussed with a Social Security representative to determine the exact requirements for individual situations.

Age at Disability	Credits Required	Age at Disability	Credits Required
31 through 42	20	52	30
44	22	54	32
46	24	56	34
48	26	58	36
50	28	60	38
		62 or older	40

End Stage Renal Disease (ESRD) Eligibility

People of any age with permanent kidney failure who receive dialysis or a kidney transplant and meet any one of the following conditions are eligible for Medicare benefits:

- You are already receiving Social Security benefits or Railroad Retirement Board benefits.

- You have worked long enough in a federal, state, or local government job to qualify.

- You are the spouse or dependent of someone who meets the eligibility requirements.

Medicare eligibility begins three months after the month in which a patient begins dialysis. Patients participating in self-dialysis training and transplant patients may be eligible sooner. Coverage can begin in the first month of dialysis if you meet the following conditions:

- You must take part in a self-dialysis training program given by a Medicare approved facility.

- You must begin the training before the third month after the dialysis begins.

- You must expect to finish the training and practice self-dialysis on a continuing basis.

If you are a transplant patient, Medicare's coverage can begin in the same month you are admitted to the hospital either for the transplant or for the preliminary testing and procedures. To qualify, the transplant must take place either in the same month or in the two months following. If the transplant is delayed beyond this time frame, your coverage will be effective two months before the month in which the transplant takes place.

Individual cases vary and therefore eligibility should be carefully checked with a Social Security representative.

◤ *Coverage Limitations*

If you have Medicare coverage only because you have permanent kidney failure and (not by reason of age or other disability) your Medicare coverage ends based on the following schedule:

- 12 months after the last dialysis treatment

- 36 months after the month in which the kidney transplant was performed

Coverage can be reinstated under any one of the following conditions:

- You resume dialysis treatment within 1 year after the month you stopped dialysis

- You resume (or begin) dialysis within 36 months after a transplant

- You receive another transplant within 36 months.

◤ *Applying for End Stage Renal Disease (ESRD) Benefits*

To apply for benefits, contact your Social Security office. You will need to provide proof of your medical condition and evidence of sufficient quarterly work credits through either your own or someone else's employment history.

DEPARTMENT OF HEALTH AND HUMAN SERVICES
Health Care Financing Administration

FORM APPROVED
OMB NO. 0938-0080

**APPLICATION FOR HEALTH INSURANCE BENEFITS
UNDER MEDICARE FOR INDIVIDUAL
WITH CHRONIC RENAL DISEASE**

I hereby request that my right to health insurance benefits be determined under Section 226 (A) of the Social Security Act.

1.	Print Your Full Name *(First name, middle initial, last name)*	Enter your Social Security Number

2. Check (✓) whether you are: ☐ Male ☐ Female

Enter your maiden name *(if applicable)*

3. Enter your date of birth (Month, day, year) ——▶

4. (a) Have you received regularly scheduled dialysis? ——▶
   (If "Yes" answer (b).)
   (If "No," go to 6.)
   ☐ Yes ☐ No

   (b) Enter beginning date(s) and ending date(s) (if applicable) of all periods of regularly scheduled dialysis *(month, year)* ——▶
   Dialysis Began: | Ended:

5. (a) Have you participated (or do you expect to participate) in a self-dialysis training program?——▶
   (If "Yes" answer (b).)
   (If "No," go to 6.)
   ☐ Yes ☐ No

   (b) Enter date self-dialysis training began (or is expected to begin) *(month, year)* ——▶

6. (a) Have you received a kidney transplant? ——▶
   (If "Yes" answer (b).)
   (If "No," go to (e).)
   ☐ Yes ☐ No

   (b) Enter date(s) of transplant(s) *(month, year)*——▶

   (c) Were you in a hospital for transplant surgery or for necessary procedures preliminary to transplant before the month you actually received the transplant?——▶
   (If "Yes" answer (d).)
   (If "No," go to 7.)
   ☐ Yes ☐ No

   (d) Enter dates of hospitalization for 6(c) *(month, day, year)* ——▶
   From: | To:

   (e) If you are scheduled to receive a transplant, enter date *(month, year)* ——▶

Form HCFA-43 (8-81) Page 1

Application for End Stage Renal Disease Patients, Page 1

7.	ENROLLMENT IN THE SUPPLEMENTARY MEDICAL INSURANCE PLAN: The medical insurance benefits plan pays for most of the costs of physicians' and surgeons' services, and other covered medical services such as OUTPATIENT MAINTENANCE DIALYSIS TREATMENTS, which are not covered by the hospital insurance plan. This plan covers outpatient treatment provided in a hospital or a facility which meets prescribed conditions. It also COVERS HOME DIALYSIS, including the rental or purchase of home dialysis machine, and the purchase of disposable equipment and supplies needed for the dialysis.		

ENROLLMENT IN THE SUPPLEMENTARY MEDICAL INSURANCE PLAN: The medical insurance benefits plan pays for most of the costs of physicians' and surgeons' services, and other covered medical services such as OUTPATIENT MAINTENANCE DIALYSIS TREATMENTS, which are not covered by the hospital insurance plan. This plan covers outpatient treatment provided in a hospital or a facility which meets prescribed conditions. It also COVERS HOME DIALYSIS, including the rental or purchase of home dialysis machine, and the purchase of disposable equipment and supplies needed for the dialysis.

Coverage under this SUPPLEMENTARY MEDICAL INSURANCE PLAN does not apply to most medical expenses incurred outside the United States. Your social security district office will be glad to explain the details of the plan and give you a leaflet which explains what services are covered and how payment is made under the plan.

Once you are enrolled in this plan, you will have to pay a monthly premium to cover part of the cost of your medical insurance protection. The Federal Government contributes an equal amount or more toward the cost of your insurance. Premiums will be deducted from any monthly social security, railroad retirement, or civil service benefit checks you receive. If you do not receive such benefits, you will be notified about when, where, and how to pay your premiums.

YOU WILL BE AUTOMATICALLY ENROLLED IN THIS PLAN UNLESS YOU INDICATE, BY CHECKING THE "NO" BLOCK BELOW, THAT YOU DO NOT WANT TO BE ENROLLED.

(a) DO YOU WISH TO ENROLL IN THE SUPPLEMENTARY MEDICAL INSURANCE PLAN? (If "No," go to 8.) ☐ Yes ☐ No

(b) If your application is processed within 5 months after the first month in which you meet all the requirements for your Medicare entitlement, your coverage will begin with that first month.

If your application is processed more than 5 months after your first possible month of entitlement, you may choose one of the following for your first month of coverage. (Please check one):

*The earliest possible month of entitlement, if you are willing and able to pay all premiums for past months of coverage ☐
OR
*The month in which this application is filed, if it is the same as, or later than, your first possible month of entitlement ☐
OR
*The month in which this enrollment will be processed ☐

ITEMS 8 THROUGH 16 REQUEST INFORMATION NEEDED TO DETERMINE INSURED STATUS FOR MEDICARE ENTITLEMENT.

8.	(a) Have you (or has someone on your behalf) ever filed an application for social security benefits, a period of disability under social security, or hospital or medical insurance under Medicare? (If "Yes," answer (b) and (c).) (If "No," go to 9.)	☐ Yes ☐ No
	(b) Enter name of person(s) on whose social security record(s) you filed other application(s)	*(First, middle initial, last)*
	(c) Enter social security number(s) of person(s) named in (b). *(If unknown, so indicate.)*	
9.	(a) Have you (or has someone on your behalf) ever filed an application for monthly benefits or hospital or medical insurance under Medicare with the Railroad Retirement Board? (If "Yes," answer (b) and (c).) (If "No," go to 10.)	☐ Yes ☐ No
	(b) Enter the name of person(s) on whose railroad record you filed other application(s)	*(First, middle initial, last)*
	(c) Enter Railroad Number of person named in (b). *(If unknown, so indicate.)*	

Form HCFA-43 (8-81) (Page 2)

Application for End Stage Renal Disease Patients, Page 2

IF YOU ARE ALREADY ENTITLED TO A MONTHLY SOCIAL SECURITY BENEFIT OR A MONTHLY RAILROAD ANNUITY, DO NOT COMPLETE ITEMS 10 THROUGH 16.

10. (a) Were you in the active military or naval service (including Reserve or National Guard active duty or active duty for training) after September 7, 1939? ⟶ ☐ Yes ☐ No

(If "Yes," answer (b).) (If "No," go to 11.)

(b) Enter dates of service ⟶

FROM:	TO:
(Month, year)	*(Month, year)*

11. Have you worked in the railroad industry any time on or after January 1, 1937? ⟶ ☐ Yes ☐ No

12.
- Enter below the names and addresses of all the persons, companies, or Government agencies for whom you worked during the last 12 months.
- If you worked in agricultural employment, give this information for this year and last year.
- If neither of the above applies, write "None" below and go to 14.

Name and address of employer *(If you had more than one employer, please list them in order beginning with your last (most recent) employer.)*	Work began		Work ended *(If still working, show "Not Ended")*	
	Month	Year	Month	Year

(If you need more space, use "Remarks" space on back page.)

13. May we ask your employers for wage information needed to process your claim? ⟶ ☐ Yes ☐ No

14. (a) Were you self-employed this year, last year, or the year before? *(If "Yes," answer (b).) (If "No," go to 15.)* ⟶ ☐ Yes ☐ No

(b) Check the year or years in which you were self-employed	In what kind of trade or business where you self-employed? *(For example, storekeeper, farmer, physician)*	Were your net earnings from your trade or business $400 or more? *(Check "Yes" or "No")*	
☐ This year			
☐ Last year		☐ Yes	☐ No
☐ Year before last		☐ Yes	☐ No

Form HCFA-43 (8-81) (Page 3)

Application for End Stage Renal Disease Patients, Page 3

IF YOU HAVE BEEN CONTINUALLY EMPLOYED FOR 2 OR MORE YEARS IN THE LAST 3 YEARS, DO NOT COMPLETE ITEMS 15 AND 16.

15. (a) Check your Marital Status. *(If single, go to 16.)*

☐ MARRIED   ☐ WIDOWED   ☐ DIVORCED   ☐ SINGLE

(b) Enter your wife's maiden name or your husband's name	Date of Birth	Date of marriage	Date of divorce (if divorced)	Date of death (If deceased)	Your wife's or your husband's Social Security or Railroad Number (If none or unknown, so indicate.)

(c) Check (✓) whether your marriage was performed by:
     ☐ Clergyman or authorized public official, or   ☐ Other *(Explain in Remarks)*

(d) Were you married before your present marriage?
(If "Yes," give the following information about each of your previous marriages. If you need more space, use "Remarks" section below or attach a separate sheet.)   ☐ Yes   ☐ No

YOUR PREVIOUS MARRIAGE	To Whom Married	When (Month, day, year)	Where (Enter name of city & State)
	How Married Ended	When (Month, day, year)	Where (Enter name of city & State)

16. Complete the following if you are single.

MOTHER'S NAME	DATE OF BIRTH	MOTHER'S SOCIAL SECURITY OR RAILROAD NUMBER
FATHER'S NAME	DATE OF BIRTH	FATHER'S SOCIAL SECURITY OR RAILROAD NUMBER

REMARKS:

IMPORTANT: Medicare coverage based on kidney failure will end with either:
     a. The last day of the 36th month after the month in which a kidney transplant is received, or
     b. The last day of the 12th month after the month in which a regular course of dialysis is discontinued, unless another course of dialysis is initiated or another transplant is received before the last day of coverage.

I AGREE TO NOTIFY THE SOCIAL SECURITY ADMINISTRATION IF THE COURSE OF DIALYSIS ENDS OR A KIDNEY TRANSPLANT IS RECEIVED.

I know that anyone who makes or causes to be made a false statement or representation of material act in an application or for use in determining a right to payment under the Social Security Act commits a crime punishable under Federal law by fine, imprisonment or both. I affirm that all information I have given in this document is true.

SIGNATURE OF APPLICANT	Date (Month, day, year)
Signature *(First name, middle initial, last name) (Write in ink)* SIGN ▶ HERE	Telephone number(s) at which you may be contacted during the day

Mailing Address *(Number and street, Apt. No., P.O. Box, or Rural Route)*

City and State	ZIP Code	Enter Name of County (if any) in which you now live

Witnesses are required ONLY if this application has been signed by mark (X) above. If signed by mark (X), two witnesses to the signing who know the applicant must sign below, giving their full addresses.

1. Signature of Witness	2. Signature of Witness
Address *(Number, Street, City, State, and ZIP Code)*	Address (Number, Street, City, State, and ZIP Code)

Form HCFA-43 (8-81) (Page 4)   ☆U.S. Government Printing Office: 1985-539-766

Application for End Stage Renal Disease Patients, Page 4

Special Situations

In certain circumstances, disabled people under 65 — children, widows and widowers, and divorced widows and widowers — can qualify for Medicare coverage based on the record of a parent, spouse, or ex-spouse. The same is true for dialysis and transplant patients. Check with Social Security on the specific details of your situation.

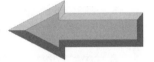

Frequently Asked Questions

Q. If I am already receiving Social Security disability payments, do I have to apply for Medicare disability benefits?

A. No. You will be automatically enrolled after you receive Social Security disability benefits for 24 months and you should receive notification of that. If you do not receive any notice of enrollment, check with Social Security. You will be subject to any waiting period in effect for receiving benefits, but you should not have to complete any additional paperwork.

Q. I receive dialysis treatment for kidney failure. How do I get Medicare benefits to help pay for the treatments?

A. You must apply. Contact your local Social Security office for an application or to make an appointment to fill out the required forms.

Q. I am on temporary disability leave from my company. Can I get Medicare disability benefits?

A. No. To qualify for Medicare disability you must be totally and permanently disabled.

Q. If I meet the definition of disability for my company's insurance plan, will I meet Medicare's requirements?

A. One does not affect the other. You will have to apply for Medicare disability benefits to find out if you qualify under Medicare's definition.

Q. I am 66 and have recently become disabled. Should I apply for Medicare disability benefits?

A. No. Disability coverage is for people who are under 65 and not yet able to apply for Medicare. If you are already receiving Medicare benefits, there would be no change in the benefits you receive. If you are not receiving Medicare benefits, you are eligible to apply for the regular Medicare coverage available to those over 65.

Q. My daughter is being treated for kidney failure. Could she be eligible for Medicare coverage?

A. Yes. If you have sufficient work credits, your dependent may be eligible for Medicare coverage for ESRD treatment. She also may be eligible based on her own work record. Contact your Social Security office for more information.

Q. Does Medicare use the same definition of disability that Social Security does?

A. Yes. The definition is very strict. Basically, you must not be able to engage in any gainful employment.

Q. I have been denied Medicare coverage for the disabled. Do I have any options?

A. First, find out why and get it in writing. If it is an error that is easily fixed such as proving your work credit history, contact Social Security and provide them with the documentation needed. If it is a question of the extent and permanence of your disability, you will probably need an attorney or other professional advocate to pursue it. Disability law is very complex and you need someone experienced in it and in how Medicare determines disability. Agencies who aid the disabled may be able to provide information about the availability of legal and advocacy services in your area.

Q. **Is there a waiting period before receiving Medicare disability coverage?**

A. Yes. There is a five-month waiting period after meeting the eligibility requirements. This waiting period starts at the time that you have met the requirement of being disabled for 24 months, so it is really a total of 29 months before benefits start.

Q. **Do I need Part B coverage if I have Medicare for ESRD?**

A. Yes. Most kidney failure related expenses are Part B expenses.

Q. **I am a dialysis patient eligible for Medicare. When will my benefits start?**

A. Three months after the month in which you begin dialysis. This waiting period can be shortened by fulfilling the self-dialysis training requirements. Check with Social Security if self-dialysis is a possibility for your treatment.

Q. **When do benefits begin for a kidney transplant?**

A. The month you enter the hospital for the transplant. It may also begin in the month you enter the hospital for medical care preliminary to a transplant, but to qualify your transplant must occur within two months.

SECTION II
TRADITIONAL MEDICARE

CHAPTER 5

Medicare Part A and Part B

Medicare Basics

Most people have both Medicare Part A and Medicare Part B coverage. This combination provides all the coverage that is available under Medicare. The two parts of the Medicare program are intended to work together to give participants a broad range of coverage, although it is not total coverage. Why Medicare is structured as two separate programs is not clear, as certainly one comprehensive plan would be more easily understood by those covered.

Medicare, at its best, is intended to help pay for medical care; it does not promise to pay for all medical care. For instance, it does not cover outpatient prescription costs, which can be substantial. And Medicare, as with all insurance carriers, reserves the right to define the care that it will cover. Just because a patient wants a certain type of treatment and/or a doctor prescribes it does not automatically mean that it will be a covered expense. All medical procedures and treatments are subject to Medicare's approval, which is why it is imperative to understand the ins and outs of the program.

In conversation, people generally do not differentiate between the two types of coverage when discussing Medicare, and this causes a great deal of misunderstanding. Medicare Part A and Medicare Part B not only are responsible for different types of expenses, they also are subject to different types of deductibles, co-payments, and other benefit limitations. In effect, it is as if you had two different insurance companies. It is crucial to understand the differences if you are ever going to make sense out of the program.

Medical Necessity

With respect to all Medicare coverage, the medical care must be medically necessary. Medically necessary means that the care must be considered appropriate for the treatment of your medical condition based on the usual standards applied by the health care profession. The determination is usually made by your attending physician, but is subject to acceptance by Medicare. Medicare will not cover any services not considered medically necessary. And, generally, it will not pay for any care that is not considered mainstream or medically proven to be beneficial. This is why most "alternative" types of health care, such as acupuncture, are not covered. Experimental procedures generally are not covered either.

If Medicare refuses to pay for something because they judged it not medically necessary, you can appeal the decision. (How to do this is discussed in Chapter 7.)

Part A Coverage

We begin with an explanation of Medicare Part A benefits, also referred to as Medicare Hospitalization Insurance. This is the basic coverage that all Medicare recipients have. The following table (see next page) offers a

Medicare Part A: 1998

Services	Benefit	Medicare Pays	Patient's Responsibility
HOSPITALIZATION Semiprivate room and board, general nursing and other hospital services and supplies.	First 60 days	All but $764	$764
	61st to 90th day	All but $191 a day	$191 a day
	91st to 150th day *	All but $382 a day	$382 a day
	Beyond 150 days	Nothing	All costs
SKILLED NURSING FACILITY CARE Semiprivate room and board, skilled nursing and rehabilitative services and other services and supplies.	First 20 days	100% of approved amount	Nothing
	Additional 80 days	All but $95.50 a day	Up to $95.50 a day
	Beyond 100 days	Nothing	All costs
HOME HEALTH CARE Part-time or intermittent skilled care, home health aide services, durable medical equipment and supplies and other services.	Unlimited as long as you meet Medicare conditions.	100% of approved amount; 80% of approved amount for durable medical equipment.	Nothing for services; 20% of approved amount for durable medical equipment.
HOSPICE CARE Pain relief, symptom management and support services for the terminally ill.	For as long as doctor certifies need.	All but limited costs for outpatient drugs and inpatient respite care.	Limited costs for outpatient drugs and inpatient respite care.
BLOOD When furnished by a hospital or skilled nursing facility during a covered stay.	Unlimited if medically necessary.	All but first 3 pints per calendar year.	For first 3 pints.

All payments are subject to the restrictions imposed by Benefit Periods.   * Assumes the use of lifetime reserve days.

glimpse at how quickly a patient's out-of-pocket costs can escalate after 60 days of hospital care. The table also shows that there are limitations to the total number of days for which Medicare will reimburse costs.

Benefit Periods

As the chart on page 66 shows, certain covered services are subject to limitations based on Benefit Periods. For Medicare Part A, a Benefit Period begins on the first day you enter a hospital and it ends when you have been out of the facility for 60 uninterrupted days.

Costs associated with re-admission to the hospital or to a skilled nursing facility within the 60-day period are considered part of the same Benefit Period. If you are admitted again within the 60 days, you are still in the same Benefit Period, even if it is the 59th day. In other words, the clock is still ticking on your remaining days of coverage.

At the end of 60 days, if you have not been readmitted to a hospital or other facility, the Benefit Period ends. If you are hospitalized on the 61st day or after, your benefits are calculated and paid as if you had not been previously hospitalized. You will be responsible for a new deductible and your co-insurance payments will begin anew at a lower daily amount.

When is a Hospital Cost Not a Hospital Cost?

The short answer about Medicare Part A is that it covers medically necessary inpatient care in a general hospital, a psychiatric hospital, a skilled nursing facility, and/or medically necessary hospice or home health care.

This appears reasonably comprehensive, but what does it really mean? To most people, for instance, this would seem to cover any expense incurred while hospitalized. Yet Part A does not pay for the doctors who attend you in the hospital, or for specialists such as anesthesiologists, psychiatrists, or surgeons. Nor does it pay for long-term care, such as that provided in a nursing home or intermediate care facility.

It seems a closer look at that simple explanation is called for. Let's review the coverage for each basic type of Medicare Part A covered services.

General Hospitalization

During an approved hospital admission Medicare will help pay for the following inpatient hospital services:

- Semiprivate room (two or more beds)

- Meals received in the hospital, including any special dietary requirements

- General medical and surgical nursing care

- Special unit nursing care (intensive care, cardiac care, etc.)

- Rehabilitation services, such as physical therapy, occupational therapy, and speech therapy

- Prescription drugs

- Medical supplies

- Lab tests

- X-rays and radiotherapy

- Blood transfusions, except for the first three pints

- Operating and recovery room charges

- Other medically necessary services and supplies

For an expense to be covered by Medicare:

- A physician must prescribe the care.

- The treatment can only be provided in a hospital.

- The hospital must participate in the Medicare program.

- The treatment cannot have been denied by a PRO (Peer Review Organization) or Medicare Intermediary.

◤ *Limitations and Benefit Periods*

There is no lifetime limitation on the number of Benefit Periods allowed for each Medicare recipient. Within each Benefit Period, the patient is responsible for a deductible and for daily co-payments that increase as the hospital stay lengthens. Medicare benefits for any single Benefit Period run out after 90 days, unless the patient has available lifetime reserve days to use. Every person enrolled in Part A has a lifetime reserve of 60 days for inpatient hospital care.

Skilled Nursing Facilities

Skilled nursing facilities are not the same as nursing homes, assisted care facilities, or intermediate care facilities, although one location may incorporate all three types of services. Skilled nursing facilities can be part of a hospital complex, or entirely separate.

A skilled nursing facility offers nursing and/or rehabilitation services that are medically necessary to a patient's recovery.

The key distinction to understand is that the services provided are not custodial in nature. In Medicare parlance, custodial services are those which basically assist a patient with personal needs, such as dressing, eating, bathing, and getting in and out of bed. Medicare will not pay for these and similar services. An exception is made when these services are included as part of the necessary daily medical care being provided on an inpatient basis, where they are a routine and necessary adjunct to the medical care.

In a skilled nursing facility, Medicare will cover:

- Semiprivate room (two or more beds to a room)

- Meals, including special dietary requirements

- Rehabilitation services, such as physical and occupational therapy

- Prescription drugs

- Other medically necessary services and supplies

To be covered, the patient must:

- Require daily skilled care which can only be provided as an inpatient in this type of facility

- Be certified by a doctor or appropriate medical professional as requiring these services on a daily inpatient basis

- Have been a hospital inpatient for at least three consecutive days before admission to the skilled nursing facility

- Be treated for the same illness or condition for which he/she was a patient in the hospital

- Be admitted within 30 days of discharge from the hospital

▰ *Limitations and Benefit Periods*

Coverage in a skilled nursing facility is limited to a maximum of 100 days per Benefit Period. The patient is responsible for daily co-payments after the 20th day. Care must be related to a hospital admission of at least three days duration.

Home Health Care

A number of services which were previously covered by Part A are being transferred to Part B coverage. This switch from one to the other is to be phased in over six years until all Home Health care services which are not related to a stay in a Skilled Nursing Facility or a hospital will be paid for under Part B.

Home health care services are provided through licensed public or private organizations that are Medicare approved. The services are generally provided by a visiting nurse or a home health care aide and are medically necessary services, not personal care or housekeeping services. Medicare approval of the home health care agency means that the organization meets certain Medicare standards necessary for reimbursement. It does not signify any type of warranty of the individuals performing the services.

The type of home health care services available are:

- Nursing services (registered and practical nurses)
- Physical therapy
- Speech therapy
- Occupational therapy

71

- Home Health Aide services

- Other medically necessary services for ongoing care

- Medical Social Services

- Durable medical equipment (e.g., hospital beds and wheelchairs) and medical supplies (e.g., bandages and splints)

With respect to the list above, patients need to know that under the provisions of the Balance Budget Act of 1997, home health care services and supplies will be gradually transferred to Part B coverage over the next six years. At the end of the six year period, the only home health care that will be covered under Part A will be 100 days of care required as the result of an in-patient or skilled nursing facility stay. Your Home Health Care Agency will be able to give you the specifics of whether Part A or Part B applies to your situation.

To qualify for Medicare reimbursement:

- The patient must be confined to the home.

- A physician must certify the medical necessity and must prescribe the program of care.

- The services must be provided by a participating Medicare home health care organization.

Home health care benefits are not for custodial care— where a patient has difficulty living on his/her own and performing daily tasks. Home health care is for medical care such as physical therapy or skilled nursing care required for monitoring the patient's progress. The distinction controls whether the patient receives coverage for the services, supplies, and equipment.

◤ *Limitations and Benefit Periods*

There are no Benefit Periods, deductibles, or co-payments required for Medicare approved home health care services. There are limitations on the maximum number of visits per week and the maximum number of hours per day that a patient can receive skilled nursing services and home health aide service.

Generally, the total number of hours for both home health aide and nursing services combined cannot exceed 28 hours per week or be more than 8 hours in a day. This insures that home health care will qualify as either "intermittent" or "part-time" care. Under certain circumstances, the number of hours can be increased to 35 per week. But this increase in hours can only be for a short period of time and must be approved by Medicare and requested by your doctor.

Psychiatric Hospitalization

Payment for inpatient psychiatric care is very limited in duration, but during the course of covered treatment the types of charges allowed are similar to those of a regular hospital.

Medicare coverage for inpatient psychiatric care covers:

- Semiprivate room (two or more beds)
- Meals received in the hospital, including any special dietary requirements
- Nursing care
- Rehabilitation services, such as physical therapy, occupational therapy, and speech therapy

73

- Prescription drugs dispensed during the hospital stay
- Medical supplies
- Lab tests
- X-rays and radiotherapy
- Blood transfusions, except for the first three pints
- Other medically necessary services and supplies

To be covered:

- A physician must prescribe the care
- The treatment can only be provided by a hospital
- The hospital must participate in the Medicare program
- The care cannot have been denied by a PRO (Peer Review Organization) or Medicare intermediary

◤ Limitations and Benefit Periods

Medicare benefits for treatment in a psychiatric hospital are limited to a lifetime maximum of 190 days. If you receive psychiatric care in addition to other medical treatment as part of a regular hospital stay, this limitation does not apply. Deductibles and co-payments are the same as for a regular inpatient hospital stay.

Hospice Care

Hospice care is care for terminally ill patients. Special provisions of the Medicare hospice care program allow for the payment of some expenses not ordinarily covered by Medicare, such as homemaker services.

Hospice care includes:

- Physician services

- Nursing care

- Prescription drugs, subject to a nominal co-pay

- Medical social services

- Home health aide and homemaker services

- Physical therapy

- Occupational therapy

- Speech therapy

- Dietary and other counseling

- Short-term respite care of up to five consecutive days (inpatient respite care allows time off for the person who regularly provides care in the home)

- Medical supplies

To qualify for payment by Medicare:

- The terminal nature of the patient's illness must be certified by a physician and the hospice Medical Director.

- The anticipated life expectancy must be six months or less.

- The patient must choose to use hospice care benefits rather than regular Medicare coverage for the treatment of the terminal illness. (The usual Medicare coverage is still available for medical expenses not related to the terminal illness.)

- The care must be provided by a hospice care agency that is approved by Medicare.

▰ *Limitations and Benefit Periods*

A hospice care patient is eligible for two 90-day Benefit Periods followed by an unlimited number of 60 day extensions. Your physician must certify the terminal nature of your illness at the beginning of the first 90 day period, and again at the beginning of each 60 day period. If the patient chooses to do so, s/he may discontinue participation in the hospice care program and switch back to regular Medicare coverage.

There are no deductibles under the hospice care program, but there is a co-pay for prescription drugs of five percent of the cost or $5 per prescription, whichever is less. There is also a co-payment for inpatient respite care of five percent of the Medicare approved rate.

In one of the Medicare system's many quirks, it should be noted that the reimbursement under the hospice provisions apply only to treatment of the terminal illness. Medical treatment for other conditions will be paid based on the usual Part A and Part B provisions.

Medicare Part B

The worst is over. Medicare Part B coverage is much easier to understand. First of all, it does not matter where you receive the services — at home, in a hospital, in a doctor's office, or in some other medical facility. Also, all costs are subject to the same deductible and the same co-insurance payments in any calendar year. The Benefit Period is the calendar year.

Medicare Part B covers:

- Outpatient hospital services
- Doctor bills

- X-rays and lab tests
- Ambulance transportation
- Breast prostheses after a mastectomy
- Physical therapy
- Occupational therapy
- Speech therapy
- Home health care (costs not covered by Part A)
- Blood transfusions, except for the first three pints
- Mammograms and Pap tests
- Outpatient mental health services
- Artificial limbs and eyes
- Arm, leg, and neck braces
- Durable medical equipment (e.g., walkers, wheelchairs, oxygen equipment)
- Kidney dialysis and kidney transplants
- Heart and liver transplants under limited circumstances
- Medical supplies (e.g., surgical dressings and casts)
- Preventive Care: screening for prostate cancer, colorectal cancer, mammography and breast exams, pap smears and pelvic exams, bone-mass density loss; flu and pneumonia inoculations; hepatitis B vaccinations.
- Some oral anti-cancer drugs and certain drugs for hospice patients

Medicare Part B: 1998

Services	Benefit	Medicare Pays *	Patient's Responsibility *
MEDICAL EXPENSES Doctors' services, inpatient and outpatient medical and surgical services and supplies, physical and speech therapy, diagnostic tests, durable medical equipment and other services.	Unlimited if medically necessary.	80% of approved amount. Reduced to 50% for most outpatient mental health services.	20% of approved amount and limited charges above approved amount.
CLINICAL LABORATORY SERVICES Blood tests, urinalyses, and more.	Unlimited if medically necessary.	Generally 100% of approved amount.	Nothing for services.
HOME HEALTH CARE Part-time or intermittent skilled care, home health aide services, durable medical equipment and supplies and other services.	Unlimited as long as you meet Medicare conditions.	100% of approved amount; 80% of approved amount for durable medical equipment.	Nothing for services; 20% of approved amount for durable medical equipment.
OUTPATIENT HOSPITAL TREATMENT Services for the diagnosis or treatment of illness or injury.	Unlimited if medically necessary.	Medicare payment to hospital based on hospital cost.	20% of whatever the hospital charges.
BLOOD	Unlimited if medically necessary.	80% of approved amount (starting with 4th pint).	First 3 pints plus 20% of approved amount for additional pints.
AMBULATORY SURGICAL SERVICES	Unlimited if medically necessary.	80% of pre-determined amount.	20% of pre-determined amount.

* All payments are subject to the $100 annual deductible.

The Basics

Medicare Part B requires payment by the patient of a $100 deductible in each calendar year. This deductible is calculated against the Medicare approved amount, which can be different from the amount billed by your doctor or other medical provider.

After satisfying the requirements of the deductible, Medicare will pay for 80 percent of the approved charges. You are responsible for the remaining 20 percent as a co-payment.

◤ Exceptions

Certain preventive screening procedures (e.g., mammograms and pap smears) and preventive inoculations (e.g., flu shots) are not subject to the Part B deductible and/or the 20% co-insurance payment.

The chart at left summarizes Part B's coverage.

Ifs, Ands, or Buts

Seems simple, right? Well, there can be complications. If Medicare does not allow any part of the charge or Medicare's approved amount is lower than the actual amount billed, you may be responsible for that amount or a portion of it. Also, some types of expenses, such as prescription drugs, are not covered at all, and the patient is responsible for all of the costs.

Exactly how much you may be responsible for depends upon a number of factors.

- If your physician or provider is a participating physician or provider, then you will only be responsible for your annual deductible and the

79

20 percent co-payment. Participating providers agree to accept Medicare's decision for the approved amount.

- If your physician or provider is not a participating provider, you will be responsible for the deductible, 20 percent co-payment, and a portion of the amount disallowed by Medicare. The amount above the 20 percent co-payment and deductible is limited to a specific percentage above the Medicare approved amount. This amount is calculated by Medicare and will appear on your EOMB form. The next chapter will explain in more detail how to understand your financial responsibility on a claim.

- If the claim is rejected in its entirety, *and* you had reason to know that the expense was not likely to be paid by Medicare, you may be responsible for the entire amount. If s/he knows that reimbursement for a claim is doubtful, your physician is required to notify you in advance in writing.

Frequently Asked Questions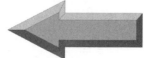

Q. **Where can I get application forms and more information about Medicare?**

A. Contact any Social Security office. The local office will be listed in the phone book.

Q. **What does Medicare Part A and Part B cover?**

A. Medicare has two parts: Hospital Insurance (Part A) and Medical Insurance (Part B).

Part A helps pay for approved charges for inpatient care in a hospital or skilled nursing facility, or for care from a home health agency or hospice.

Part B helps pay for physician services, outpatient hospital care, clinical laboratory tests, and various other medical services and supplies, including durable medical equipment.

Q. What is a Part A Benefit Period?

A. A Part A Benefit Period begins the day you are hospitalized and ends after you have been out of the hospital or skilled nursing facility for 60 consecutive days, or if you remain in a skilled nursing facility but do not receive any skilled care there for 60 days in a row. There is no limit to the number of Benefit Periods you can have in a lifetime.

Q. How much are the Part B deductible and co-insurance amounts?

A. In 1998, the Medicare Part B deductible is $100 per year. You are responsible for the first $100 of approved expenses for physician and other medical services and supplies per year. After you have met the annual deductible, then Medicare generally pays 80 percent of all other approved charges for covered services for the rest of the year. You are responsible for the other 20 percent co-payment. There is no deductible or co-insurance for home health services.

Q. How much are the Part A deductible and co-insurance amounts for hospital stays?

A. The Part A deductible is $764 per Benefit Period in 1998. Medicare then pays all approved expenses for the first 60 days. The Part A deductible applies to each Benefit Period, so it is possible that you may have to pay more than one deductible in a year if you are hospitalized more than once.

In each Benefit Period, Medicare pays all approved expenses except for a co-insurance amount of $191 per day (in 1998) for days 61 to 90 of hospitalization. If more than 90 days of inpatient hospital care are needed in a Benefit Period, you can use some or all of your lifetime reserve days to pay for covered services. Every person enrolled in Part A has a lifetime reserve of 60 days for inpatient hospital care. Once used, these days are not renewed. When a reserve day is used, Medicare pays for all covered services except for a co-insurance amount ($382 a day in 1998).

Q. **Who pays for the co-insurance and deductibles?**

A. The patient is responsible for deductibles and co-insurance payments. If s/he has a Medigap policy, the policy will cover some of these costs.

Q. **What if I am sent to a skilled nursing facility after leaving the hospital?**

A. If, after being in a hospital for at least three days, you require approved care in a skilled nursing facility, Part A will help cover services for up to 100 days per Benefit Period. Medicare pays all covered expenses for the first 20 days and all but $95.50 per day (in 1998) for the next 80 days. After 100 days in any Benefit Period, Medicare pays nothing.

Q. **What doesn't Medicare pay for?**

A. Custodial care (except during hospice care), eyeglasses, hearing aids, eye exams, hearing exams, telephone, TV, or radios used during a hospital stay, most outpatient prescription drugs, non-prescription medicines, cosmetic surgery, most immunizations, dental care, routine foot care, and routine physical checkups. And, of course, the deductibles and co-payments.

Q. Does Medicare cover ambulance services?

A. Yes, under certain conditions Part B will pay when: (1) the ambulance, equipment, and personnel meet Medicare requirements; and (2) transportation by any other means would endanger your health.

Q. Does Medicare cover artificial limbs?

A. Yes. They must be provided by a hospital, skilled nursing facility, home health agency, hospice, comprehensive outpatient rehabilitation facility (CORP), or a rural health clinic.

Q. What kind of medical supplies or durable medical goods will Medicare pay for?

A. Medicare covers cardiac pacemakers, corrective lenses needed after cataract surgery, colostomy or ileostomy supplies, breast prostheses following a mastectomy, and artificial limbs and eyes. Durable medical equipment covered includes wheelchairs, hospital beds, walkers, and other equipment prescribed by a doctor for home use.

Q. Does Medicare provide coverage for mammograms?

A. Yes. Medicare Part B will pay for annual mammograms and the payment is not subject to the Part B deductible.

Q. Does Medicare pay for pap smears?

A. Yes, and also for pelvic exams. Payment will be made for pap smears and pelvic exams on an every three year basis. For women who are at high risk of vaginal or uterine cancer, this coverage may be extended to be done annual basis.

Q. Does Medicare pay for care in a psychiatric hospital?

A. Yes. Medicare Part A helps pay for up to 190 days of inpatient care in a participating psychiatric hospital. The 190 days of care is a lifetime maximum. Once used, it is not renewed.

Q. Does Medicare cover home health care?

A. Yes, if it is medically required for the treatment of an illness or injury as determined by your physician. The services must be provided by a participating home health care agency, you must be homebound, and you must need part-time or intermittent skilled nursing care, physical therapy, or speech therapy. Your physician must also provide a plan of care.

Q. How long will Medicare cover home health care?

A. There is no time limitation, provided the services are covered services and are provided by a participating Medicare provider. Continued reimbursement is dependent upon your physician's determination of the services you require and Medicare's approval. There are limitations on the number of visits per week for skilled nurses and home health aides.

Q. How much will Medicare cover for the costs of home health care?

A. For Part A expenses, Medicare pays the full approved cost of all home health care visits and there is no co-insurance. You will be charged a 20 percent co-insurance payment of the approved costs of any durable medical equipment required. For expenses under Part B, you must pay the annual deductible and the 20 percent co-insurance payment.

Q. What is hospice care?

A. Hospice care is care for terminally ill patients whose life expectancy is six months or less.

Q. Does Medicare cover hospice care?

A. Yes, if the patient is certified by a physician to be terminally ill.

Q. Does my managed care plan pay for hospice care?

A. No. Hospice care is paid through traditional Medicare.

Q. What are the Benefit Periods for hospice care?

A. Medicare has special Benefit Periods for those patients who are in the hospice program. There are two 90 day Benefit Periods, followed by an unlimited number of 60 day Benefit Periods.

Q. If I am traveling or residing outside the United States and its territories, will Medicare cover my medical expenses?

A. Only if you are treated in a qualified Canadian or Mexican hospital and meet one of the following three conditions:

1. You are in the United States when an emergency occurs, and a Canadian or Mexican hospital is closer to your location than the nearest U.S. hospital.

2. You live in the United States, and a Canadian or Mexican hospital is closer to your home than the nearest U.S. hospital that can provide the care required even if it is not an emergency situation.

3. You are in Canada traveling by the most direct route between Alaska and another state when an emergency occurs, and a Canadian hospital is closer to your location than the nearest U.S. hospital that can provide the emergency treatment.

Under any other circumstances, Medicare will not cover your expenses.

CHAPTER 6

Understanding
Medicare Claims

The Good News

You don't file Medicare claims, your doctor, hospital, or health care provider does. This is true even for fee-for-service patients.

Several years ago, Congress decided that one of the ways to control Medicare costs was to have all claims filed in a similar manner and hopefully, at some future date, electronically. So, Congress mandated that medical service providers, including doctors, must file Medicare claims directly from their offices for all their Medicare patients. This attempt at cost control actually had a decidedly beneficial effect for consumers.

It eliminated a great deal of paperwork for Medicare recipients. If you have a Medigap policy, that claim is often filed with your Medigap insurer for you by the Medicare Carrier after they have processed the original claim. This eliminates the Medigap claim paperwork for you.

How the Claim Process Works

In most instances (there are very infrequent exceptions), the beginning of the claim filing process will be out of your hands. The details that follow show how, in the best of all worlds, it will work. This does not mean that you can sit back and relax about your claim processing. You will still need to be aware of the submissions made on your behalf and track the payments received. This is necessary to ensure that a mistake has not been made, that a prompt appeal can be filed if necessary, and to understand your obligations regarding payments you need to make.

As with everything else about Medicare, Part A and Part B transactions are handled slightly differently.

◢ Part A Claims

Billing for services that are Part A expenses is done directly between the provider and the Medicare intermediary. The patient is not responsible for filing this claim and should not be billed by the provider before Medicare reviews the claim. A hospital may ask the patient to pay the deductible and any non-covered expenses at the time of discharge. After making a determination on the claim, Medicare will send the patient a statement called a Medicare Benefit Notice (see next page).

This form carries a prominent notice stating: "This is not a bill." And it isn't. The form contains information about the action which Medicare took regarding the claim. It will indicate:

- The name of the person or organization who furnished the medical services

- The dates on which the services were rendered

- The date of the notice

- The claim number

- The Medicare benefits that were used in payment of the claim

U.S. DEPARTMENT OF HEALTH AND HUMAN SERVICES / HEALTH CARE FINANCING ADMINISTRATION

MEDICARE BENEFIT NOTICE

220012   **DATE:** 10 / 01 / 96

JANE SMITH
1500 E. 64TH ST.
NEW YORK, NY   55555

HEALTH INSURANCE CLAIM NUMBER
999999999A

Always use this number
when writing about your claim

THIS IS NOT A BILL

This notice shows what benefits were used by you and the covered services not paid by Medicare for the period shown in item 1. See other side of this form for additional information which may apply to your claim.

1 SERVICES FURNISHED BY	DATE(S)	BENEFITS USED
CAPE COD HOSPITAL 27 PARK ST HYANNIS MA 02601	09 / 09 / 96 THRU 09 / 11 / 96	2 INPATIENT HOSPITAL DAYS

2 PAYMENT STATUS	PAID DATE: 10 / 03 / 96

MEDICARE PAID ALL COVERED SERVICES.

IF NO-FAULT INSURANCE, LIABILITY INSURANCE, WORKERS' COMPENSATION,
DEPARTMENT OF VETERANS AFFAIRS, OR, IN SOME CASES, A GROUP HEALTH PLAN
FOR EMPLOYEES ALSO COVERS THESE SERVICES, A REFUND MAY BE DUE THE MEDICARE
PROGRAM. PLEASE CONTACT US IF YOU ARE COVERED BY ANY OF THESE SOURCES.
YOU DO NOT HAVE TO CONTACT US TO REPORT A MEDICARE SUPPLEMENTAL (MEDIGAP)
POLICY.

THE FLU SEASON IS APPROACHING. NOW IS A GOOD TIME TO MAKE PLANS FOR YOUR
ANNUAL FLU SHOT. PLEASE REMEMBER THAT FLU SHOTS ARE NOW COVERED BY MEDICARE.

C&S ADMINISTRATIVE SERVICES
P.O. BOX 2194
BOSTON   MA   02106
1-800-882-1228

If your have any questions
about this record, call
or write

(outside of Massachusetts)
1-617-741-3300

TELEPHONE NUMBER

Medicare Benefits Notice

- The amount, if any, that the patient is responsible for paying

- The phone number and address of the Medicare intermediary that processed the claim

If the patient is responsible for a payment, the notice will state the amount and the reason (e.g., deductible) for the balance due. No payment should be made from this statement; the patient will be billed separately by the provider for the charges indicated, if they have not already been paid.

◤ Part B Claims

Part B claims are a bit more confusing to the patient. The provider is still responsible for billing Medicare, but there are a number of possible variations. For instance, the provider may or may not be a participating provider and s/he may or may not accept assignment. Both situations influence the amount that the patient needs to pay.

In general, when a patient seeks treatment from a doctor or other medical provider s/he will give his/her Medicare identification number to the provider. The provider will probably make a copy of the patient's Medicare card as well. After treating the patient, the provider will bill Medicare on behalf of the patient. If the patient pays the provider at the time of service, Medicare will send the reimbursement to the patient. If the provider has not been paid by the patient, Medicare will pay the provider directly.

In either situation, Medicare will send a notification to the patient, an Explanation of Medicare Benefits (EOMB) form (see following pages). This form has the same purpose as the Medicare Benefits Notice which is sent after review of Part A

THIS IS NOT A BILL
Explanation of Your Medicare **Part B** Benefits

JANE SMITH
1500 E. 64TH ST.
NEW YORK   NY   55555

Summary of this notice date August 31, 1996		
Total Charges:	$	510.00
Total Medicare approved:	$	296.48
We paid your provider:	$	237.18
Your total responsibility:	$	59.30

Your Medicare Number is : 999-99-9999A

Your provider <u>accepted</u> assignment

Details about this notice (See the back for more information.)

BILL SUBMITTED BY:
Mailing Address:

MEDICAL ANESTHESIOLOGISTS
Church St. Station, New York, NY 10249

Dates	Services and Service Codes	Charges	Medicare Approved	See Notes Below
	Control number 94230-6058-00-000			b
	DR. JOHN JONES			
Aug. 10, 1996	1 Anesth, hip joint surgery (01210-AA)	$ 510.00	$ 296.48	a

Notes:

a   The approved amount is based on the fee schedule.
b   This information is being sent to your private insurer.

GENERAL INFORMATION ABOUT MEDICARE

The flu season is approaching. Now is a good time to make plans for your annual flu shot. Please remember that flu shots are now covered by Medicare.

(continued on next page)

**IMPORTANT: If you have questions about this notice, call Medicare at (516) 244-5100 (toll free 1-800-442-8430) or see us at 122 East 42nd Street, 3rd Floor New York, N.Y. You will ned this notice if you contact us.
To appeal our decision, you must WRITE to us before MAR. 3, 1997 at Medicare Part B, P.O. BOX 2280, Peekskill, NY 10566-0991. See #2 on the back.**   (000-0100120)

Explanation of Medicare Benefits, Page 1

Page 2

JANE SMITH

Your Medicare Number is :999-99-9999A

More details about this notice

Here's an explanation of this notice:

Of the total charges, Medicare approved	$	296.48	The provider agreed to accept this amount.
Your 20%	–	59.30	We pay 80% of the approved amount; you pay 20%.
The 80% Medicare pays	$	237.18	**You have already met the deductible for 1996.**
Medicare owes	$	237.18	
We are paying the provider	$	237.18	
Of the approved amount	$	296.48	
Less what Medicare owes	–	237.18	
Your total responsibility	$	59.30	The provider may bill you for this amount. If you have other insurance, the other insurance may pay this amount.

IMPORTANT: If you have questions about this notice, call Medicare at (516) 244-5100 (toll free 1-800-442-8430) or see us at 122 East 42nd Street, 3rd Floor New York, N.Y. You will ned this notice if you contact us.
To appeal our decision, you must WRITE to us before MAR. 3, 1997 at Medicare Part B,
P.O. BOX 2280, Peekskill, NY 10566-0991. See #2 on the back. (000-0100120)

Explanation of Medicare Benefits, Page 2

claims. The similarity stops there. An EOMB form looks different and is more complicated to read and understand.

The EOMB is a very important document and it provides a lot of information. It will tell the patient:

- The name of the physician or provider who submitted the claim.

- The date or dates of medical service.

- The type of service provided.

- How much Medicare was billed for the service.

- How much Medicare approved for payment.

- Who was paid (the provider or the patient). If the patient is being paid, there will be a check enclosed with the EOMB form.

- An explanation of Medicare's payment, including information about deductible, co-insurance, and charges that were not allowed.

- The additional amount the patient must pay to the provider.

- The phone number and address of the Medicare carrier who processed the claim.

- Whether a Medigap insurance claim also was forwarded to your Medigap insurer.

After reviewing the EOMB form, you will know exactly what Medicare paid and how much you owe to the medical provider. The amount on the EOMB form is the total amount you should pay to a provider—that is all you owe on the claim covered.

Keeping Track of Medical Claims

It is important to keep track of medical claims filed and paid. Mistakes do happen and sometimes providers bill a patient for more than they are entitled to collect. Also, the total amount due from a patient is not always readily apparent at the time the service is rendered. A provider may ask for payment of co-insurance or deductible amounts at the time of the service. This is based on the fee s/he expects to receive from Medicare. It may or may not be accurate. The only way to protect against overpaying a provider on a claim is to be aware of and fully understand Medicare's claim decision and to keep a log of all payments made by Medicare, the patient, and any other insurance carriers involved, such as Medigap.

Never assume that a bill or statement sent to you from the provider is correct. The last line item on an EOMB form states the total amount you are responsible for paying. If you have been billed for more than that or have paid more than that, you need to contact the provider. If possible, try to pay your provider after you have seen the EOMB form, which will make it easier for you to compare the bill with the amount on the EOMB form.

With respect to following the progress of claims through the system, a few items are important to note. We've highlighted areas on the EOMB form to show where to find the information needed.

- Always reference a claim by the date of service, not the date the claim form was printed. The date of service is the date of the doctor's appointment or the date medical service was provided. You will find the date of service on the EOMB form.

Provider's name

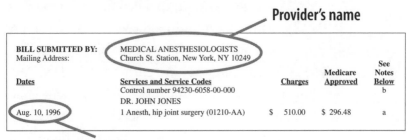

BILL SUBMITTED BY:	MEDICAL ANESTHESIOLOGISTS			
Mailing Address:	Church St. Station, New York, NY 10249			
			Medicare	See Notes
Dates	**Services and Service Codes**	**Charges**	**Approved**	**Below**
	Control number 94230-6058-00-000			b
	DR. JOHN JONES			
Aug. 10, 1996	1 Anesth, hip joint surgery (01210-AA)	$ 510.00	$ 296.48	a

Date of service

- The provider's name that appears on the EOMB can sometimes be misleading because it may not match the name of the provider or doctor as you know it. For instance, doctors who are part of a group practice may file with Medicare under the group's name, not their own names. Sometimes Medicare inputs the wrong doctor's name when there are several on the claim form. When this occurs, it can be confusing. If you are not certain what the charge is for, check with the Medicare carrier or check with the doctor or provider you saw on the referenced date of service.

- Note to whom payment was made by Medicare, either the provider or you. If to you, a check will be enclosed with the EOMB form. The check amount needs to be reconciled with any money you have paid directly to the provider to see if there is any balance due to the provider or if there has been an overpayment.

- Note how much was billed by the provider and how much Medicare approved. This is important to you, as the Medicare approved amount determines the payments from Medigap policies and also limits your costs.

Approved amount

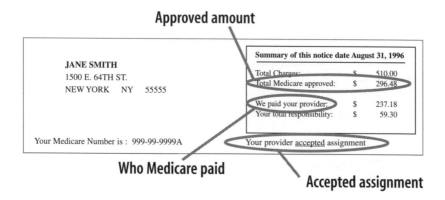

JANE SMITH
1500 E. 64TH ST.
NEW YORK   NY   55555

Summary of this notice date August 31, 1996

Total Charges:	$	510.00
Total Medicare approved:	$	296.48
We paid your provider:	$	237.18
Your total responsibility:	$	59.30

Your Medicare Number is : 999-99-9999A

Your provider accepted assignment

Who Medicare paid

Accepted assignment

■ Check whether the provider accepted assignment from Medicare. If so, then you are only responsible for the 20 percent co-payment and any remaining annual deductible.

■ See what your total out-of-pocket responsibility is. This is indicated in the summary section shown below and again on the last line of the form.

■ Determine whether you have met the annual deductible or if it is included in the amount you are responsible for paying.

Annual deductible

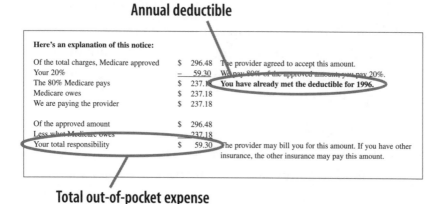

Here's an explanation of this notice:

Of the total charges, Medicare approved	$	296.48	The provider agreed to accept this amount.
Your 20%	−	59.30	We pay 80% of the approved amount; you pay 20%.
The 80% Medicare pays	$	237.18	You have already met the deductible for 1996.
Medicare owes	$	237.18	
We are paying the provider	$	237.18	
Of the approved amount	$	296.48	
Less what Medicare owes		237.18	
Your total responsibility	$	59.30	The provider may bill you for this amount. If you have other insurance, the other insurance may pay this amount.

Total out-of-pocket expense

Dates	Services and Service Codes	Charges	Medicare Approved	See Notes Below
	Control number 94230-6058-00-000			b
	DR. JOHN JONES			
Aug. 10, 1996	1 Anesth, hip joint surgery (01210-AA)	$ 510.00	$ 296.48	a

Notes:

a   The approved amount is based on the fee schedule.
b   This information is being sent to your private insurer.

Explanation   **Reference code**

- Note the explanation for the rejection or reduction of any charges. Medicare's explanations are referenced by line item. If you do not agree, you have the option of appealing the decision.

- If you have a Medigap policy, check to see if the claim has already been forwarded to that carrier for payment. In some states, the claims are filed automatically. In other states, the patient must file the claim with the Medigap company after receiving the EOMB form.

All the information you need is available on the EOMB form. After reviewing a few forms, they will be easier to understand. Matching the information on the EOMB form with bills you receive from providers and with the payments you have made is time-consuming and often tedious work. And, if you have follow-up questions or you want to appeal a decision, the time commitment can grow. It is important to follow through on these items, though, because costs can mount quickly and no one should pay more than is necessary.

If you have a few claims in a year, you can probably keep track of what you owe and to whom with relatively little fuss. You just need to compare any payments you have made to the provider or have been billed for by the provider with the information on the EOMB form.

Date of Service	Provider Name	Amount Billed to Medicare	Amount Paid by Medicare	Balance Remaining	Amount Billed to Medigap*	Amount Paid by Medigap	Amount Owed by Patient	Date Paid in Full *	Amount Paid by Patient
					* or other insurance company			* claim complete	

With severe or long-term illnesses the large number of claims that are submitted can become a nightmare. Nothing is going to make it easy, but keeping track of the paperwork from the beginning can reduce the total time spent and reduce the possibility of overpayments or duplicate payments.

To know what your bottom line is, you will need to know what Medicare paid, what you have paid, and what your Medigap carrier has paid (if you have one). A form similar to the one shown on page 97 will give you the information needed. It can be adjusted to your particular situation and is easily done by hand or on a computer.

Using a format similar to the one shown will allow you to keep track of the paperwork for each claim.

Frequently Asked Questions

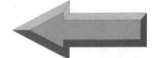

Q. How do I file a Medicare claim?

A. You don't, except on rare occasions. Under federal law, the medical care provider must file the claim for you. And in many states, the claim will automatically be referred to your Medigap carrier, if you have one. If for some reason you have to file a claim directly, call your Medicare carrier (see list in Appendix A) and ask for instructions.

Q. Who processes Medicare claims and payments?

A. Insurance companies who have a contract with the federal government to do so. The organizations handling claims from hospitals, skilled nursing facilities, home health agencies, and hospices are called "intermediaries." The organizations that handle Medicare's Part B claims are called "carriers." Sometimes the same organization handles both Part A and Part B claims, but you will still receive separate notices. The names and addresses of the intermediaries and carriers along with the locations they serve are listed in Appendix A and are available from any Social Security Administration office.

Q. How does Medicare decide on an approved amount for medical services?

A. Medicare's system of payment is not easily understood by the patient. In essence, Medicare has developed a system that reflects average costs for various treatments and conditions and it pays based on those numbers.

There is a uniform national system for designating diagnoses and treatments. Each service or diagnosis has a specific number assigned to it which Medicare references when processing the claim. Medicare pays claims based on the approved cost associated with a particular code number and diagnosis.

This coding is important because a mistake can cause a claim to be rejected or not paid in full. Many claims will have multiple codes and more than one diagnosis written down. In order to work within the system, the provider must include all the appropriate codes.

Q. If I have a question about a Medicare claim for a doctor's services who do I call?

A. Doctors' services are Part B expenses so call the Medicare carrier for your area. The name and toll-free phone number will appear on the Explanation of Medicare Benefits (EOMB) form that covers the claim in question. There is

99

also a list of all carriers in Appendix A or you can contact Social Security and ask for the phone number.

Q. How long should I wait before contacting the Medicare carrier to check on the status of a claim?

A. If you have not received a Medicare Benefits Notice or an Explanation of Medicare Benefits (EOMB) payment statement within 45 days of filing the claim, call the Medicare carrier for your area. There are strict time frames within which Medicare must respond to a claim, but bear in mind that the provider may not have filed the claim immediately. Make sure you have your Medicare number available before you call.

Q. I think Medicare did not allow the proper amount in payment of a claim. What do I do?

A. You will have to file an appeal of Medicare's decision. Follow the procedures outlined in the next chapter.

Q. I received a Medicare Benefit Notice which showed that all costs associated with my hospitalization had been paid except for my deductible. Why am I also getting bills from the surgeon and my regular physician if all costs have been paid?

A. All Part A costs were paid, but fees from surgeons and medical doctors are Part B expenses even though they treated you while in the hospital. The doctors involved should have filed separate claims with Medicare Part B if you have that coverage. Call their offices and ask them to hold the bills until you receive your EOMB form. If you do not have Medicare Part B coverage (or other insurance), you are liable for the costs as out-of-pocket expenses.

Q. I keep receiving bills for more than the amount that my EOMB form says I owe to the doctor. What should I do?

A. Contact the doctor's office and tell them you are not liable for more than the amount on the EOMB form. Send them a copy of the form if necessary and ask them to bill you for the corrected amount. This happens more often than it should, so it is important to keep clear records as to the status of claims.

Q. My doctor is a participating doctor. What does that mean?

A. Participating doctors agree to accept Medicare's approved amount as their fee for services rendered. This means they will not bill you for additional costs if Medicare finds that the fee they billed is more than the Medicare approved cost. The patient is still responsible for the annual deductible and the 20 percent co-insurance amount. The deductible and co-insurance payments will be based on the approved amount, not the actual charge from the doctor.

Q. My doctor is not a participating physician. Is it possible that s/he will accept assignment anyway?

A. Yes. Any physician or provider can decide to accept assignment. S/he can accept assignment on one claim, a series of claims pertaining to the same illness, or for all claims. Discuss this with your provider before beginning treatment. Also, some states require providers to accept assignment on all charges related to Medicare claims.

Q. How do I know whether my state requires doctors to be participating providers?

A. You can either call your state insurance office and ask them (see Appendix D for phone numbers) or you can call the

Medicare Carrier for your state (see Appendix A). Either source should be able to give you the information.

Q. My Medigap policy covers my deductible and co-insurance payments. Will my doctor file a claim for me?

A. Some doctors will, so you should ask your doctor. Otherwise, just attach a copy of your EOMB form to the claim form for your Medigap carrier; this will usually be sufficient for processing the claim.

In some states, the Medicare carrier will process the Medigap claim at the same time. Your EOMB form will state if the Medigap claim was sent to your Medigap insurer.

Q. My doctor keeps billing me for more than the amount for which I am responsible even though I sent his office a copy of the EOMB. What do I do?

A. Contact the doctor again. If you still receive bills in the wrong amount, contact the Medicare carrier listed on the EOMB and ask for assistance. If this fails, call the Office of the Inspector General at (800) 368-5779 and ask for assistance. Keep copies of all your correspondence.

CHAPTER 7

Appealing Medicare Decisions

You Have a Right to Appeal

Medicare isn't always right. There are specific ways to appeal any Medicare decision and you have every right to question a decision. Even though it can be intimidating to "fight back" when it comes to the government, an appeal of a decision you believe is wrong is often decided in your favor, particularly with appeals of medical claim decisions.

Unfortunately for patients, decisions about medical care are no longer simply a matter of discussion between doctor and patient. In this cost-conscious age, there are additional layers of evaluations to go through to make certain your costs are covered. The review process is negotiated between your physician or hospital and Medicare. All this oversight can lead to conflicting opinions about medical necessity, and places a great deal of pressure on the patient's physician to make a solid case for the need for treatment.

How Medicare Decides on Approved Costs

Before delving into the specifics of how to appeal a claim, we need to explain the basis that Medicare uses for making claims decisions. Contrary to what we may think at times, there is a basis on which Medicare determines its approved costs for various types of medical treatment. This does not mean that Medicare never makes mistakes, so do not accept a determination that seems to be unfair or in conflict with your coverage.

Anyone who has lived in more than one region of the country knows that there can be a wide variation in the cost of coverage for the same medical treatment, in New York versus Iowa, for example. There may also be a variation in the way treatment is handled, the length of hospital stays, and how often a particular type of treatment is ordered.

This variation can have many reasons, including the availability of up-to-date medical facilities and the expertise of the people providing treatment. Medicine is often referred to as an art, not a science, which means that you are buying a qualified opinion from your medical provider, and that opinion may vary from someone else's.

In order to bring coherence and some degree of consistency to the processing of hospital related medical claims, Medicare uses a system based on peer review organizations (PROs). Peer review organizations are groups of doctors hired by Medicare to evaluate different types of treatments. The idea is to combine Medicare's concerns for cost containment with the medical community's expertise in determining the necessity of various treatments.

Medicare allows PROs to decide issues such as the necessity for hospital admission for different illnesses, the appropriate length of stay in a hospital or skilled nursing facility for specific illnesses and procedures, the review of hospital admission decisions, re-admissions and discharges, and approval of home health care or hospice care.

In effect, the PROs develop "typical" guidelines for medical care procedures so Medicare can use this information for processing claims, and to aid Medicare in eliminating coverage for unnecessary medical treatment. The PROs also review treatment prescribed in specific cases to determine whether it should be covered by Medicare as medically necessary.

The issues of cost containment and medical necessity can often be at odds, however, and guidelines are just that. They need to be tempered by evaluation of individual needs, and it is quite possible that the PRO's decision about specific care can be at odds with your own physician's decision. This can lead to a situation where you feel it is necessary to appeal a Medicare decision.

Each PRO is under contract to Medicare; one PRO usually covers a whole state or a large portion of it. We provide the list of PROs by state in Appendix C.

In addition to the PROs, which cover many facilities, individual hospitals each have a committee of doctors known as the utilization review committee (URC). URCs review the use of services and care in their own hospital. Their decisions are supposed to be made without regard to who is paying for the care, be it Medicare, the patient, or another insurance company, and the decisions are supposed to be made based on medical criteria. But in the real world these physicians are under pressure by the hospitals to control costs. Their decisions about your case may be open to question because all decisions are ultimately subjective in nature.

Also, to confuse the issue even more, the hospital's URC may have been designated by a PRO to function in the place of the PRO. In this situation, the URC is acting under the assumption that Medicare will be responsible for the payment for approved care, and the decisions are related to meeting Medicare's needs and directives about cost containment.

Payments made for Part B expenses are based on the Medicare Fee Schedule. This schedule is arrived at by breaking all procedures down into their component parts and assigning a value to them. The dollar value arrived at is then adjusted for differences in geographic location. Only the computer nerds at Medicare could possibly explain the ins and outs of this calculation.

If this isn't enough bureaucracy, the Medicare carrier and intermediary organizations that process the claims also have a say in whether a cost is justified. These organizations are responsible for reviewing the information provided about a patient's condition and deciding whether or not Medicare will approve the treatment costs. In deciding to accept or reject charges, they essentially perform a type of medical review. In that respect, they overlap the function of the PROs and URCs.

What to Do If You Disagree

If you disagree with a Medicare claim decision, by all means question it. As a patient, you have nothing to lose and everything to gain. The odds are good that at some point you will disagree with the way Medicare has handled a claim for services.

Medicare's decisions are based on a lot of averages—average number of days of treatment, average cost for treatment, average recovery time, and so forth. Your case may not be average.

There are a variety of reasons for Medicare to reject a charge. The key to a successful appeal is finding out exactly why coverage is being denied and who made the decision. Then you can work with your physician to address the specific difficulty.

The information provided about appealing a decision will familiarize you with the steps in the process. There are many variables among cases, but this chapter will provide you with the basic information about how to proceed. As with everything else about Medicare, the appeals process is different for Part A and Part B claims.

Appealing a Part A Claim

◤ *Hospital claims*

If you are denied Medicare coverage for a hospital admission or for charges relating to an inpatient stay, you have the right to appeal the decision.

There are any number of reasons why coverage may be denied: the hospital may have been denied Medicare payment in a similar situation; or the PRO may feel that the treatment is necessary, but can be performed on an outpatient basis; or the surgery can be handled at an ambulatory surgery center at a lower cost; or that you should be sufficiently recovered to go home. Whatever the reason, get it in writing.

All PRO determinations made regarding hospital care are supposed to be strictly related to medical necessity and the circumstances of the particular situation. All Medicare hospital patients should be given a written copy of their "bill of rights" when admitted (see following page). This notice spells out the patient's rights and the format for contesting a decision.

If a hospital denies you admission or decides that you should be discharged earlier than you believe advisable, and the decision has been made by the hospital utilization review

---

AN IMPORTANT MESSAGE FROM MEDICARE

YOUR RIGHTS WHILE YOU ARE A MEDICARE HOSPITAL PATIENT

- You have the right to receive all the hospital care that is necessary for the proper diagnosis and treatment of your illness or injury. According to Federal law, **your discharge date must be determined solely by your medical needs**, not by "DRGs" or Medicare payments.

- You have the right to be fully informed about decisions affecting your Medicare coverage and payment for your hospital stay and for any post-hospital services.

- You have the right to request a review by a Peer Review Organization of any written Notice of Noncoverage that you receive from the hospital stating that Medicare will no longer pay for your hospital care. Peer Review Organizations (PROs) are groups of doctors who are paid by the Federal Government to review medical necessity, appropriateness and quality of hospital treatment furnished to Medicare patients. The phone number and address of the PRO for your area are:

_____

_____

_____

TALK TO YOUR DOCTOR ABOUT YOUR STAY IN THE HOSPITAL

You and your doctor know more about your condition and your health needs than anyone else. Decisions about your medical treatment should be made between you and your doctor. **If you have any questions about your medical treatment, your need for continued hospital care, your discharge, or your need for possible post-hospital care, don't hesitate to ask your doctor.** The hospital's patient representative or social worker will also help you with your questions and concerns about hospital services.

IF YOU THINK YOU ARE BEING ASKED TO LEAVE THE HOSPITAL TOO SOON

- Ask a hospital representative for a written notice of explanation immediately, if you have not already received one. This notice is called a "Notice of Noncoverage." You must have this Notice of Noncoverage if you wish to exercise your right to request a review by the PRO.

- The Notice of Noncoverage will state either that your doctor or the PRO agrees with the hospital's decision that Medicare will no longer pay for your hospital care.

  —If the hospital and your doctor agree, the PRO does not review your case before a Notice of Noncoverage is issued. But the PRO will respond to your request for a review of your Notice of Noncoverage and seek your opinion. You cannot be made to pay for your hospital care until the PRO makes its decision, if you request the review by noon of the first work day after you receive the Notice of Noncoverage.

Patient's "Bill of Rights," Page 1

—If the hospital and your doctor disagree, the hospital may request the PRO to review your case. If it does make such a request, the hospital is required to send you a notice to that effect. In this situation the PRO must agree with the hospital or the hospital cannot issue a Notice of Noncoverage. You may request that the PRO reconsider your case after you receive a Notice of Noncoverage but since the PRO has already reviewed your case once, you may have to pay for **at least one day of hospital care** before the PRO completes this reconsideration.

IF YOU **DO NOT** REQUEST A REVIEW, **THE HOSPITAL MAY BILL YOU** FOR ALL THE COSTS OF YOUR STAY BEGINNING WITH THE THIRD DAY AFTER YOU RECEIVE THE NOTICE OF NONCOVERAGE. THE HOSPITAL, HOWEVER, CANNOT CHARGE YOU FOR CARE UNLESS IT PROVIDES YOU WITH A NOTICE OF NONCOVERAGE.

HOW TO REQUEST A REVIEW OF THE NOTICE OF NONCOVERAGE

- If the Notice of Noncoverage states that your **physician agrees** with the hospital's decision:

  —You must make your request for review to the PRO by **noon of the first work day** after you receive the Notice of Noncoverage by contacting the PRO by phone or in writing.

  —The PRO must ask for your views about your case before making its decision. The PRO will inform you by phone and in writing of its decision on the review.

  —If the PRO agrees with the Notice of Noncoverage, you may be billed for all costs of your stay beginning at noon of the day **after** you receive the PRO's decision.

  —Thus, you will **not** be responsible for the cost of hospital care before you receive the PRO's decision.

- If the Notice of Noncoverage states that the PRO agrees with the hospital's decision:

  —You should make your request for reconsideration to the PRO **immediately** upon receipt of the Notice of Noncoverage by contacting the PRO by phone or in writing.

  —The PRO can take up to three working days from receipt of your request to complete the review. The PRO will inform you in writing of its decision on the review.

  —Since the PRO has already reviewed your case once, prior to the issuance of the Notice of Noncoverage, the hospital is permitted to begin billing you for the cost of your stay beginning with the third calendar day after you receive your Notice of Noncoverage **even if the PRO has not completed its review**.

  —Thus, if the PRO continues to agree with the Notice of Noncoverage, **you may have to pay for at least one day of hospital care**.

NOTE: The process described above is called "immediate review." If you miss the deadline for this immediate review while you are in the hospital, you may still request a review of Medicare's decision to no longer pay for your care at any point during your hospital stay or after you have left the hospital. The Notice of Noncoverage will tell you how to request this review.

Patient's "Bill of Rights," Page 2

committee (URC) without involving the PRO, you may request a review of the decision by the PRO. This request may be made via telephone or in writing to the PRO. In this situation the URC is acting on behalf of the hospital, not Medicare. The PRO acts for Medicare and its decision is called a determination. Only a determination may be appealed.

If the determination by the PRO is not favorable you may begin the formal appeals process, which has three parts:

- Request for reconsideration by the PRO

- Request for a hearing before an Administrative Law Judge

- Request for a hearing before the Appeals Council

You must go through each stage in the above order. The initial request for reconsideration can be made by you, by your doctor, or by the hospital. The request for a hearing must be made by you (or someone you choose as your representative). In the latter case, it is advisable to retain the services of a professional advocate or attorney who is knowledgeable about the Medicare appeals process.

The formal appeals process starts with the filing of form HCFA-2649, a Request for Reconsideration of Part A Health Insurance Benefits form. This form may be filed by you, or if you are an inpatient, the hospital may file it on your behalf (see next page).

This request must be filed within 60 days of the notice of Medicare claim determination. If you are seeking admission to a hospital or are being discharged from a hospital, you may request expedited processing of the request which takes three days. Otherwise, the PRO has up to 30 days to issue a determination.

DEPARTMENT OF HEALTH AND HUMAN SERVICES
HEALTH CARE FINANCING ADMINISTRATION

Form Approved
OMB No. 0938-0045

REQUEST FOR RECONSIDERATION OF PART A HEALTH INSURANCE BENEFITS

INSTRUCTIONS: *Please type or print firmly.* Leave the block empty if you cannot answer it. Take or mail the WHOLE form to your Social Security office which will be glad to help you. Please read the statement on the reverse side of page 2.

1. BENEFICIARY'S NAME

2. HEALTH INSURANCE CLAIM NUMBER

3. REPRESENTATIVE'S NAME, IF APPLICABLE   (☐ RELATIVE   ☐ ATTORNEY   ☐ OTHER PERSON)   ☐ PROVIDER FILING

4. PLEASE ATTACH A COPY OF THE NOTICE(S) YOU RECEIVED ABOUT YOUR CLAIM TO THIS FORM.

5. THIS CLAIM IS FOR
☐ INPATIENT HOSPITAL   ☐ SKILLED NURSING FACILITY (SNF)   ☐ HEALTH MAINTENANCE ORGANIZATION (HMO)
☐ EMERGENCY HOSPITAL   ☐ HOME HEALTH AGENCY (HHA)

6. NAME AND ADDRESS OF PROVIDER *(Hospital, SNF, HHA, HMO)*   CITY AND STATE   PROVIDER NUMBER

7. NAME OF INTERMEDIARY   CITY AND STATE   INTERMEDIARY NUMBER

8. DATE OF ADMISSION OR START OF SERVICES   9. DATE(S) OF THE NOTICE(S) YOU RECEIVED

10. I DO NOT AGREE WITH THE DETERMINATION ON MY CLAIM. PLEASE RECONSIDER MY CLAIM BECAUSE

11. YOU MUST OBTAIN ANY EVIDENCE *(For example, a letter from a doctor)* YOU WISH TO SUBMIT
☐ I HAVE ATTACHED THE FOLLOWING EVIDENCE
☐ I WILL SEND THIS EVIDENCE WITHIN 10 DAYS
☐ I HAVE NO ADDITIONAL EVIDENCE OR OTHER INFORMATION TO SUBMIT WITH MY CLAIM

13. ONLY ONE SIGNATURE IS NEEDED. THIS FORM IS SIGNED BY
☐ BENEFICIARY   ☐ REPRESENTATIVE   ☐ PROVIDER REP

SIGN HERE ▶

14. STREET ADDRESS

12. IS THIS REQUEST FILED WITHIN 60 DAYS OF YOUR NOTICE?
☐ YES ☐ NO
IF YOU CHECKED "NO" ATTACH AN EXPLANATION OF THE REASON FOR THE DELAY TO THIS FORM

CITY, STATE, ZIP CODE

TELEPHONE   DATE

15. If this request is signed by mark (X), TWO WITNESSES who know the person requesting reconsideration must sign in the space provided on the reverse side of this page of the form.

DO NOT FILL IN BELOW THIS LINE—FOR SOCIAL SECURITY USE—THANK YOU

16. ROUTING
☐ INTERMEDIARY
☐ HCFA, RO-MEDICARE
☐ BSS, ODR

18. SSA OR INTERMEDIARY DATE STAMP

17. ADDITIONAL INFORMATION

FORM **HCFA-2649** (8-79)
DESTROY PRIOR EDITIONS

Request for Reconsideration of Part A Health Insurance Benefits

If the reconsideration is not favorable to you, you may move to the next step in the process and file form HA-501.1, Request for Hearing. This form must be filed within 60 days of the Reconsideration of Determination decision and the claim or group of claims must total $200.

If, after the hearing, you are again denied coverage, you may file within 60 days for a review of the hearing decision. This is done with form HA-520, Request for Review of Hearing Decision.

The appeals process is a complicated one. It is recommended that you have advice from someone knowledgeable about the appeals process for the second and third stages of the appeals process.

In all three cases, the requirement for timely filing may be waived if you can prove there were extenuating circumstances that caused you to miss the filing deadline, such as mental or physical incapacity due to illness.

◤ Skilled Nursing Facilities, Home Health Care and Hospice Care Claims

This process is basically the same as that of hospital-related claims. The key difference is that decisions regarding care in a skilled nursing facility, home health care services, and hospice care are made by the Medicare intermediary organization, not the PRO.

Once again, it is important to understand clearly what was denied, by whom it was denied, and why.

Be sure to get a written notice of denial, so that it will be available should you wish to appeal the determination. In these cases, make certain that the medical provider has actually submitted the claim to Medicare, not just made the decision on his/her own. You can only appeal an Intermediary's denial of coverage.

Part B Appeals

Part B appeals also have three stages:

- Request for review
- Request for a hearing
- Request for an Administrative Law Judge hearing

If your doctor accepted assignment, s/he will file the appeal on your behalf. If the claim was not assigned, you will have to do the paperwork and follow-up. When you appeal a Part B claim, you are appealing the decision of the Medicare carrier responsible for processing the claim. More than 50 percent of the claims appealed are decided in the claimant's favor, so it is well worth appealing a determination you feel is incorrect.

Start with your Explanation of Medicare Benefits (EOMB) form. It will explain why Medicare made the decision it did. The next step is to contact the Medicare carrier for additional information if you do not fully understand the reason for the decision.

Understanding why the claim was denied is important in framing your request for reconsideration. The key to success is providing additional or corrected information that will allow the carrier to change its decision. Without new information it is unlikely that you will receive a more favorable determination.

You have six months from the date of the EOMB to file a request for reconsideration. Some carriers can handle this request over the phone, so start with a call to the office listed on the EOMB form. If the request cannot be resolved over the phone, you can write a letter to the carrier whose address is printed on the EOMB form, or you can use form HCFA 1964, Request for Review of Part B Medical Claim (see next page).

If you write a letter, be specific about the reason for your request and state that you are asking for a review of the claim. Be sure to include:

- Your name and address

- Your Medicare number

- The claim number from the EOMB form

- The date of the EOMB form

- The reasons why you think the decision should be changed

- Any documentation you believe will support your case (i.e., copies of medical records)

- A copy of the EOMB form so Medicare has all the information to easily identify the claim in question

If you need additional records and cannot get them, let the Medicare carrier know this. The carrier may be able to help obtain them for you. And don't hesitate to ask for help from your doctor in explaining the circumstances of your treatment to Medicare. S/he may be able to provide the additional information needed to change the decision. Medicare usually will send you a written response within 30 days.

If the reconsideration results in another denial of all or part of the claim, you may request a hearing on the review.

You can file this appeal within six months of the date of the reconsideration decision. The amount in question must be at least $100. To reach this minimum amount, you are allowed

DEPARTMENT OF HEALTH AND HUMAN SERVICES
HEALTH CARE FINANCING ADMINISTRATION

Form Approved
OMB No. 0938-0033

REQUEST FOR REVIEW OF PART B MEDICARE CLAIM
Medical Insurance Benefits - Social Security Act

NOTICE-Anyone who misrepresents or falsifies essential information requested by this form may upon conviction be subject to fine and imprisonment under Federal Law.

1 Carrier's Name and Address

2 Name of Patient

3 Health Insurance Claim Number

4 I do not agree with the determination you made on my claim as described on my Explanation of Medicare

Benefits dated:

5 MY REASONS ARE: (Attach a copy of the Explanation of Medicare Benefits, or describe the service, date of service, and physician's name–NOTE.–If the date on the Notice of Benefits mentioned in item 3 is more than six months ago, include your reason for not making this request earlier.)

6 Describe Illness or Injury:

7 ☐ I have additional evidence to submit. (Attach such evidence to this form.)

☐ I do not have additional evidence.

COMPLETE ALL OF THE INFORMATION REQUESTED. SIGN AND RETURN THE FIRST COPY AND ANY ATTACHMENTS TO THE CARRIER NAMED ABOVE. IF YOU NEED HELP, TAKE THIS AND YOUR NOTICE FROM THE CARRIER TO A SOCIAL SECURITY OFFICE, OR TO THE CARRIER. KEEP THE DUPLICATE COPY OF THIS FORM FOR YOUR RECORDS.

8

SIGNATURE OF **EITHER** THE CLAIMANT **OR** HIS REPRESENTATIVE

Representative	Claimant	
Address	Address	
City, State, and ZIP Code	City, State, and ZIP Code	
Telephone Number	Date	Telephone Number	Date

Form HCFA-1964 (8-85)

(Over)

Request for Review of Part B Medical Claim

to include more than one denied claim so that, when added together, they total $100.

The hearing is sometimes held in person, sometimes on the phone, and sometimes based solely on a review of the written record provided. You choose whether to appear before the hearing officer when you fill out the form.

If you have to take this step, try to identify the additional information that will help your appeal. You need to address the issues raised in the review process completely and carefully in order to win a change of decision. Medicare will respond within 30 days.

If the previous steps have failed, you can ask for a hearing before an administrative law judge. One claim or several claims together will have to total $500 to be considered for a hearing.

The process is similar, but this hearing officer works for the Office of Hearings and Appeals in the Social Security Administration. The hearing officer in the prior appeal stage is an employee of the Medicare carrier.

You must file form HA 501, Request for Hearing by Administrative Law Judge, within 60 days of the denial by the last hearing officer. As an alternative, you may write a letter to the last hearing officer stating that you wish to request this new hearing. The officer will forward the request to the Office of Hearings and Appeals. When filing the request, be sure to include copies of all the written denials previously received.

Frequently Asked Questions

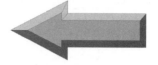

Q. I received an EOMB form denying coverage for a lab bill. What do I do?

A. Call the Medicare carrier listed and see if you can resolve the denial on the phone by providing additional information. If not, file a Request for Review of a Part B Medicare Claim, and include all relevant additional information.

Q. I want to file an appeal of a Part A claim denial, but it is more than 60 days since the determination. Is there anything I can do?

A. This depends on why you are late in filing the appeal. If you can prove that there was a true hardship that delayed the filing, Medicare may grant an exception and allow the appeal to be filed. Situations such as mental or physical disability or proof of a delay in receiving the documents needed to submit your case can result in a waiver of the time limits.

Q. I need assistance with filing a Medicare request for a hearing. Where can I get help?

A. Start by contacting the Aging Agency in your area (see listing in Appendix G) and explain the type of help you need. Ask if they can refer you to a Medicare advocacy organization or if they know of a program which provides legal services at a reduced cost.

Q. My claim for coverage was rejected because of a lack of medical necessity. What type of documentation do I need to appeal this decision?

A. You will need to convince Medicare that, in your case, the care was reasonable and necessary. To do so, you will probably need the help of your doctor and copies of your medical records. Discuss the situation with your doctor and ask for copies of any appropriate medical records to document the need for the treatment.

Q. My doctor accepted assignment, but I received an EOMB showing that coverage was denied. Do I have to appeal this?

A. No. If the provider accepted assignment, s/he will file the appeal. You are not responsible for the bill if the doctor accepted assignment.

Q. If Medicare denies coverage for a hospital stay, can my doctor still admit me?

A. Yes. If the doctor and the hospital agree that the care is medically necessary, you can be admitted. Medicare will not pay for the care (unless you appeal the decision and win), so the hospital will expect you to be responsible for all the costs. If possible, try to appeal the decision before being admitted by asking for an expedited determination.

Q. What is an expedited determination?

A. If you are seeking admission to a hospital or are being discharged from one because Medicare has rejected your claim, you can appeal this determination and ask for a speedy answer. An expedited determination will be handled in three days or less.

Q. The home health care agency says that Medicare will not pay for my claim, but has not actually submitted the bills. Is that a problem for me?

A. Yes. You can only appeal a Medicare decision once a formal determination has been made. In this case, you need the agency to submit the bills to see if Medicare really does deny the coverage. You can only appeal something that has actually been denied by the Medicare carrier. And you will need the information on your EOMB form as the basis for starting your appeal.

Q. Can I have my sister represent me during the appeals process?

A. Yes. You can choose anyone to represent you that you wish. For the purpose of handling the appeals process for you, you will need to put this in writing to Medicare and as always, there is a form, HCFA-1696, Appointment of Representative (see below). If you need a copy, call Social Security and ask them to send it to you.

DEPARTMENT OF
HEALTH AND HUMAN SERVICES
HEALTH CARE FINANCING ADMINISTRATION

NAME (Print or Type)	H.I. Claim Number

Section I   **APPOINTMENT OF REPRESENTATIVE**

I appoint this individual: _____
(Print or type name and address of individual you want to represent you.)

to act as my representative in connection with my claim or asserted right under Titles XI, or XVIII of the Social Security Act. I authorize this individual to make or give any request or notice; to present or to elicit evidence; to obtain information; and to receive any notice in connection with my claim wholly in my stead.

SIGNATURE (Beneficiary)	ADDRESS
TELEPHONE NUMBER	DATE
(Area Code)	

Section II   **ACCEPTANCE OF APPOINTMENT**

I,_____, hereby accept the above appointment. I certify that I have not been suspended or prohibited from practice before the Social Security Administration or the Health Care Financing Administration; that I am not, as a current or former officer or employee of the United States, disqualified from acting as the claimant's representative; and that I will not charge or receive any fee for the representation unless it has been authorized in accordance with the laws and regulations referred to on the reverse side hereof. In the event that I decide not to charge or collect a fee for the representation I will notify the Social Security Administration and the Health Care Financing Administration (completion of Section III (optional) satisfies this requirement).

I am a/an _____
(Attorney, union representative, relative, law student, etc.)

SIGNATURE (Representative)	ADDRESS
TELEPHONE NUMBER	DATE
(Area Code)	

Section III (Optional)   **WAIVER OF FEE OR DIRECT PAYMENT**

(Note to Representative: You may use this portion of the form to waive a fee or to waive direct payment of the fee from withheld past-due benefits.)

I waive my right to charge and collect a fee for representing _____
_____before the Social Security Administration or Health Care Financing Administration.

SIGNATURE	DATE

(See important information on reverse)

Form **HCFA-1696-U4** (10-84)

Appointment of Representative

CHAPTER **8**

Medigap Policies

What They Do

One aid to financial self-protection is the purchase of an insurance policy known as a Medigap policy. This type of policy can be purchased directly from an insurer and is also sold through various consumer groups, such as AARP. Medigap policies supplement the coverage provided under a fee-for-service Medicare plan.

These policies offer a good way to supplement Medicare Part A and Part B coverage relating to medical costs and hospitalizations. They are designed to cover items such as deductibles, co-insurance payments, and prescription drugs. They do not provide any coverage for nursing home care or other long-term custodial care options.

Medigap insurance is regulated by state and federal laws, which helps consumers compare prices. The federal government and the insurance industry developed ten standard policies. Prior to the standardization many people bought multiple Medigap policies and inadvertently purchased duplicate coverage.

Limiting the number of policy types and specifying the coverage options available in each makes it easier to comparison shop. Once you have decided on the policy or policies that best suit your needs, you simply have to compare prices and quality among the insurers.

The ten policy types are differentiated by letter. The letter A policy is the most basic coverage available and the letter J policy offers the most protection. As you proceed through the alphabet, each new letter policy contains all the coverage in Plan A (basic coverage), plus specific additional items. Thus, a D policy contains all the coverage in the letter A plan, plus various additional protections.

Not all states allow the sale of all policies, so people in some areas have fewer options than others. Within a state, however, all similarly designated policies have the same coverage no matter what insurance company is issuing the policy. Federal law prohibits an insurer from selling you more than one Medigap policy. This is a consumer protection measure to prevent paying for duplicate coverage.

Medigap Consumer Protections

Insurance companies selling Medigap policies must abide by the following regulations:

- Medigap policies must have a 30-day money-back guarantee. Once you have the policy, if it does not meet your needs you may return it within 30 days of receipt and receive a full refund.

- New Medigap policies cannot impose more than a six-month waiting period for pre-existing illnesses.

- There is a six-month open enrollment period in which you can buy a Medigap policy regardless of your health, although you may still be subject to a six-month waiting period for costs relating to pre-existing illnesses.

- Medigap policies are guaranteed renewable, unless they lapse for non-payment of premium or you made false statements on the application.

- If you switch from one Medigap policy to another and your prior Medigap policy was in effect for six months or more, payment for pre-existing illnesses cannot be restricted. There is an exception for any types of coverage under the new plan that you did not have under the old plan. For new coverage benefits only, you may have to wait up to six months.

- Insurers are prohibited from selling you a Medigap plan which duplicates Medicare coverage.

Medigap Plans

The standard plans may vary slightly state by state, but most plans adhere to the following formats. Medigap policies assume that you have both Part A and Part B coverage. Each policy provides coverage for gaps in both Parts of Medicare and you cannot buy a policy that deals with only one Part or the other.

As you will see in the following descriptions, each of the plans builds on the Basic Plan benefits that are listed under Plan A. Plan B through Plan J each include these Basic Benefits and add various additional benefits to it.

Plan A – The Basic Policy

- Coverage for the Part A co-insurance amount for the 61st through the 90th day of hospitalization in each Medicare Benefit Period.

- Coverage for the Part A co-insurance amount for each of Medicare's 60 non-renewable lifetime hospital reserve days.

- After all Medicare hospital benefits are exhausted, coverage for 100 percent of the eligible Medicare Part A hospital expenses. Coverage is limited to a maximum of 365 days of additional inpatient hospital care during the policyholder's lifetime. This benefit is paid at the Medicare approved rate.

- Coverage under Medicare Parts A and B for the reasonable cost of the first three pints of blood or equivalent quantities of packed red blood cells per calendar year unless replaced in accordance with federal regulations.

- Coverage for the co-insurance amount for Part B services (generally 20 percent of the approved amount or 50 percent of approved charges for out-patient mental health services) after $100 annual deductible is met.

Plan B

Includes all the Plan A basic benefits, plus

- Coverage for the Medicare Part A inpatient hospital deductible ($764 per Benefit Period in 1998).

Plan C

Includes all the Plan A basic benefits, plus

- Coverage for the Medicare Part A inpatient hospital deductible ($764 per Benefit Period in 1998),

- Coverage for the skilled nursing facility care co-insurance amount ($95.50 per day for days 21 through 100 per Benefit Period in 1998),

- Coverage for the Medicare Part B deductible ($100 per calendar year in 1998), and

- 80 percent coverage for medically necessary emergency care in a foreign country, after a $250 deductible.

◤ Plan D

Includes all the Plan A basic benefits, plus

- Coverage for the Medicare Part A inpatient hospital deductible ($764 per Benefit Period in 1998),

- Coverage for the skilled nursing facility care co-insurance amount ($95.50 per day for days 21 through 100 per Benefit Period in 1998),

- 80 percent coverage for medically necessary emergency care in a foreign country, after a $250 deductible, and

- Coverage for at-home recovery. The at-home recovery benefit pays up to $1600 per year for short-term assistance with activities of daily living (bathing, dressing, personal hygiene, etc.) for people recovering from an illness, injury, or surgery. There are various benefit requirements and limitations.

▰ *Plan E*

Includes all the Plan A basic benefits, plus

- Coverage for the Medicare Part A inpatient hospital deductible ($764 per Benefit Period in 1998),

- Coverage for the skilled nursing facility care co-insurance amount ($95.50 per day for days 21 through 100 per Benefit Period in 1998),

- 80 percent coverage for medically necessary emergency care in a foreign country, after a $250 deductible, and

- Coverage for preventive medical care. The preventive medical care benefit pays up to $120 per year for such items as a physical examination, serum cholesterol screening, hearing test, diabetes screening, and thyroid function test.

▰ *Plan F*

Includes all the Plan A basic benefits, plus

- Coverage for the Medicare Part A inpatient hospital deductible ($764 per Benefit Period in 1998),

- Coverage for the skilled nursing facility care co-insurance amount ($95.50 per day for days 21 through 100 per Benefit Period in 1998),

- Coverage for the Medicare Part B deductible ($100 per calendar year in 1998),

- 80 percent coverage for medically necessary emergency care in a foreign country, after a $250 deductible, and

- Coverage for 100 percent of Medicare Part B excess charges. Plan pays a specified percentage of the difference between Medicare's approved amount for Part B services and the actual charges (up to the amount of charge limitations set by either Medicare or state law).

▰ *Plan G*

Includes all the Plan A basic benefits, plus

- Coverage for the Medicare Part A inpatient hospital deductible ($764 per Benefit Period in 1998),

- Coverage for the skilled nursing facility care co-insurance amount ($95.50 per day for days 21 through 100 per Benefit Period in 1998),

- Coverage for 100 percent of Medicare Part B excess charges. Plan pays a specified percentage of the difference between Medicare's approved amount for Part B services and the actual charges (up to the amount of charge limitations set by either Medicare or state law),

- 80 percent coverage for medically necessary emergency care in a foreign country, after a $250 deductible, and

- Coverage for at-home recovery. The at-home recovery benefit pays up to $1600 per year for short-term assistance with activities of daily living (bathing, dressing, personal hygiene, etc.) for those recovering from an illness, injury, or surgery. There are various benefit requirements and limitations.

◤ Plan H

Includes all the Plan A basic benefits, plus

■ Coverage for the Medicare Part A inpatient hospital deductible ($764 per Benefit Period in 1998),

■ Coverage for the skilled nursing facility care co-insurance amount ($95.50 per day for days 21 through 100 per Benefit Period in 1998),

■ 80 percent coverage for medically necessary emergency care in a foreign country, after a $250 deductible, and

■ Coverage for 50 percent of the cost of prescription drugs up to a maximum annual benefit of $1250 after the policyholder meets a $250 per year deductible. This is called the "Basic Prescription Drug Benefit."

◤ Plan I

Includes all the Plan A basic benefits, plus

■ Coverage for the Medicare Part A inpatient hospital deductible ($764 per Benefit Period in 1998),

■ Coverage for the skilled nursing facility care co-insurance amount ($95.50 per day for days 21 through 100 per Benefit Period in 1998),

■ Coverage for 100 percent of Medicare Part B excess charges. Plan pays a specified percentage of the difference between Medicare's approved amount for Part B services and the actual charges (up to the amount of charge limitations set by either Medicare or state law),

■ Coverage for 50 percent of the cost of prescription drugs up to a maximum annual benefit of $1250 after the policyholder meets a $250 per year deductible. This is called the "Basic Prescription Drug Benefit."

■ 80 percent coverage for medically necessary emergency care in a foreign country, after a $250 deductible, and

■ Coverage for at-home recovery. The at-home recovery benefit pays up to $1600 per year for short-term assistance with activities of daily living (bathing, dressing, personal hygiene, etc.) for those recovering from an illness, injury, or surgery. There are various benefit requirements and limitations.

▰ *Plan J*

Includes all the Plan A basic benefits, plus

■ Coverage for the Medicare Part A inpatient hospital deductible ($764 per Benefit Period in 1998),

■ Coverage for the skilled nursing facility care co-insurance amount ($95.50 per day for days 21 through 100 per Benefit Period in 1998),

■ Coverage for the Medicare Part B deductible ($100 per calendar year in 1998),

■ Coverage for 100 percent of Medicare Part B excess charges. Plan pays a specified percentage of the difference between Medicare's approved amount for Part B services and the actual charges (up to the amount of charge limitations set by either Medicare or state law),

- 80 percent coverage for medically necessary emergency care in a foreign country, after a $250 deductible, and

- Coverage for 50 percent of the cost of prescription drugs up to a maximum annual benefit of $3000, after the policyholder meets a $250 per year deductible. This is called the "Extended Drug Benefit."

- Coverage for at-home recovery. The at-home recovery benefit pays up to $1600 per year for short-term assistance with activities of daily living (bathing, dressing, personal hygiene, etc.) for those recovering from an illness, injury, or surgery. There are various benefit requirements and limitations.

- Coverage for preventive medical care. The preventive medical care benefit pays up to $120 per year for such items as a physical examination, serum cholesterol screening, hearing test, diabetes screening, and thyroid function test.

The Balanced Budget Act added two new high deductible versions of Plan F and Plan J to the list of approved Medigap policy forms. They will have the same coverage as Plan F or Plan J, but they will have a $1500 per year deductible. As these high deductible versions are brand new for 1998, it may take some time for the insurance companies to begin offering them in your state.

Even with these standardized policies, it can be time consuming and a bit confusing to decide among them. Coverage does vary from state to state and not all versions of the policies may be offered.

Ten Medigap Standardized Policies
(Not all may be available in all states.)

A	B	C	D	E	F	G	H	I	J
Basic Benefit	Basic Benefit	Basic Benefit	Basic Benefit	Basic Benefit	Basic Benefit	Basic Benefit	Basic Benefit	Basic Benefit	Basic Benefit
		Skilled Nursing Coinsurance	Skilled Nursing Coinsurance	Skilled Nursing Coinsurance	Skilled Nursing Coinsurance	Skilled Nursing Coinsurance	Skilled Nursing Coinsurance	Skilled Nursing Coinsurance	Skilled Nursing Coinsurance
	Part A Deductible	Part A Deductible	Part A Deductible	Part A Deductible	Part A Deductible	Part A Deductible	Part A Deductible	Part A Deductible	Part A Deductible
		Part B Deductible			Part B Deductible				Part B Deductible
					Part B Excess (100%)	Part B Excess (100%)		Part B Excess (100%)	Part B Excess (100%)
		Foreign Travel Emergency	Foreign Travel Emergency	Foreign Travel Emergency	Foreign Travel Emergency	Foreign Travel Emergency	Foreign Travel Emergency	Foreign Travel Emergency	Foreign Travel Emergency
			At-Home Recovery			At-Home Recovery		At-Home Recovery	At-Home Recovery
							Basic Drug Benefit ($1,250 Limit)	Basic Drug Benefit ($1,250 Limit)	Extended Drug Benefit ($3,000 Limit)
				Preventive Care					Preventive Care

In some states the standard Medigap policies available may have additional benefits that are not part of these ten policy formats. Within your state, however, there are certain standard policies that are sold by all insurers to residents of that state. For instance, in Massachusetts there are only three types of Medigap policy sold and their coverage varies somewhat from the ten standard policies.

The chart at left summarizes the coverage available in the ten standard national policies.

Medicare Select

Medicare Select is a slightly different variety of Medigap policy. A recent addition, it is offered by insurance companies and some HMOs. Medicare Select policies offer the same coverage as regular Medigap policies and come in the standard plans, but there are restrictions as to which medical providers you may use.

With a standard Medigap policy you can choose any physician or other medical provider for your care, but this freedom of choice is not allowed under a Select plan. Under a Medicare Select policy you must obtain your medical care from a list of specified network doctors and providers.

If you work within the network of providers specified by the plan, you will receive full coverage for the benefits provided by your particular plan. If you seek treatment from a provider outside the plan's network, you may have to pay all or part of the charges otherwise covered by your Select policy. Medicare will still pay for its portion of the charges, but your supplemental coverage may be denied, leaving you with a bill for items such as deductibles and co-payments.

Medigap Policy Comparison Worksheet

Item	Policy 1	Policy 2	Policy 3
Company name			
A. M. Best rating			
Monthly premium			
Medigap policy type (A, B, C, etc.)			
Part A deductibles paid			
Part B deductibles paid			
Prescriptions paid			
Part A hospital co-insurance paid			
Part B co-insurance paid			
Preventive services paid			
Additional hospital days paid			
Part A skilled nursing facility co-insurance paid			
Annual or lifetime limitation on total expenses paid			
Pre-existing illness exclusions			
Other:			

This coverage option should have lower premium charges than traditional Medigap policies of the same type because of the limitations imposed regarding choice of provider.

Evaluating Medigap Options

If you are considering a Medigap policy, you need to take two steps. First, you should decide which type of policy best suits your needs (A, B, C, or whatever your state offers). Then you need to compare the costs among the numerous insurance companies who offer these policies. To help make this decision a bit clearer, use a chart like the one shown at left to evaluate your options.

Buyer Beware

A few words of advice about purchasing Medigap or any type of insurance policy:

■ Insurance agents are interested in selling policies, but their job also entails fully explaining the policy to you. Make sure you understand what you are buying.

■ Always use a check to pay for a policy. This gives you a record of payment and payment date should you decide not to keep the policy.

■ Always compare prices and coverage. This is a competitive business.

■ Don't accept comments such as "that's not a problem" or "that isn't what it really means." If the policy says it, the insurance company means it. So stick to your guns about asking questions when you are unclear about something.

133

■ Check the insurance company's A. M. Best's rating. This is a rating system that gives you information about an insurance company's financial situation and stability. Best's Insurance Reports should be available in the public library.

■ Be cautious when replacing a policy. It is important to understand exactly what the differences are between the old policy and the new one. Make certain that you are clear on what the differences are and what it will cost to switch.

Frequently Asked Questions

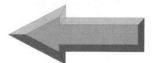

Q. What is Medigap insurance?

A. Medigap insurance is private health insurance designed specifically to supplement Medicare's benefits. It fills in some of the gaps in Medicare's Part A and Part B coverage. A Medigap policy pays for items such as deductibles, co-payments, prescription drugs, and additional inpatient hospital days.

Q. What are the gaps in Medicare coverage?

A. Among the items not paid by Medicare are deductibles and co-insurance amounts, charges in excess of Medicare's approved amounts, additional days of care in a hospital or skilled nursing facility beyond Medicare's maximums, and prescription drugs.

Q. I have a Medigap policy; do I need more than one?

A. No, and it is illegal for an insurance company to sell you more than one policy. If you want to buy additional coverage, you should upgrade your present policy by purchasing one with more comprehensive coverage. If you have two policies, you will be paying for duplicate coverage, not better coverage.

Q. How do I find out which standard policies are sold in my state?

A. Contact the Insurance Department in your state or the insurance counseling division of your state's aging agency. The locations and phone numbers are listed in Appendix D of this book.

Q. Whom should I contact if I have a complaint about someone who sold me a Medigap policy?

A. Suspected violations of the laws governing the sales and marketing of Medigap policies should be reported to your state's insurance department (see Appendix D for phone numbers and locations) or federal authorities. The federal toll-free telephone number for registering such complaints is (800) 638-6833.

Q. If I am in a Medicare HMO, do I need a Medigap policy?

A. No. This would be a duplication of coverage. Medigap policies are designed for payment of costs related to fee-for-service plans.

Q. I moved from one state to another and my new Medigap policy does not have quite the same coverage as my previous one. Can I keep the old one?

A. No. The Medigap policies may differ from state to state, but you can only buy the ones which are legal in your state.

Q. I have a Medigap policy and am thinking of switching to an HMO instead. Can I get my Medigap policy back if I don't like the HMO?

A. Yes. You can switch back to a regular Medicare program and a Medigap policy, if you wish.

Q. If I switch from an HMO to traditional Medicare coverage, are there any pre-existing illness exclusions?

A. Not with your Medicare coverage, but there might be with your supplementary coverage if you choose to purchase a Medigap policy. Check with the insurer issuing your Medigap policy.

Q. I'm switching to a new Medigap insurer to get a lower premium. Will the insurer exclude my pre-existing conditions?

A. Not if you had your other policy for six months or more and the coverage is the same. If the new policy has additional coverage that the old one did not, you may be subject to pre-existing illness limitations only on the new areas of coverage—and only for up to six months.

Q. Do Medigap policies cover nursing home care?

A. No. Medigap policies supplement Medicare coverage. They are subject to the same medically necessary standard that Medicare imposes.

Q. How does Medicare SELECT differ from Medigap?

A. It is a type of Medigap coverage which requires you to use doctors and other medical providers within a specific network. Unlike other Medigap policies, this places certain limitations on your choice of physician.

Q. **What is the benefit of buying Medicare SELECT rather than a regular Medigap policy?**

A. The premium should be lower with the SELECT policy. By limiting you to certain approved providers, the insurer has more control over costs.

SECTION III
THE NEW "IMPROVED" MEDICARE

CHAPTER **9**

Managed Care
and Medicare

Managed Care Now

Several years ago, Medicare added a limited number of managed care policies to the program both to widen the choices available to enrollees and to test the effectiveness of the plans. They were only available in some areas of the country and most of those available were of the Health Maintenance Plan (HMO) variety, which offered very limited flexibility for patients with respect to choice of doctor or other medical providers.

Approximately 13% of Medicare enrollees took advantage of these plan options and are now enrolled in some form of managed care. As you will see in the next chapter, where we discuss the new Medicare+Choice program and the changes coming in 1998 and 1999, Congress has restructured Medicare in the hope of seeing this number rise dramatically.

This chapter, however, deals with managed care in general, and the specific types of plans that now exist under Medicare. The managed care plans which are currently certified by Medicare must be re-certified in 1998 and become part of the new Medicare+Choice program. If they don't meet the new plan requirements, they will be replaced by a Medicare+Choice plan.

How Managed Care Works with Medicare

All managed care plans are not Medicare plans. Once HCFA certifies that a plan meets the Medicare coverage requirements, the agency signs a contract with the managed care organization to provide Medicare services to eligible beneficiaries. HCFA then pays the plan a monthly premium for each enrolled member. In return for these payments, the managed care plan provides you with Medicare coverage. It also may pay for Medicare deductibles or co-payments and provide additional services not covered by traditional Medicare.

To enroll in a managed care plan, you must pay the Part B premium because the managed care plan replaces both Part A and Part B coverage.

Most of the plans provide at least the coverage offered under Part A and Part B. In many instances, they also include the coverage gained by having a Medigap policy along with Part A and Part B. The plan may charge you an additional monthly premium and/or may require a small co-payment at the time services are rendered. The specifics of co-pays and premiums vary by plan and by the type of coverage provided.

Some plans also allow you to purchase additional coverage (e.g., dental, eye care, preventive care, prescriptions, etc.) which is not part of the traditional Medicare coverage.

◤ Enrollment Requirements

You may switch to a managed care plan during any enrollment period specified by the plan. All plans must have at least one 30-day open enrollment period each year. Many plans allow you to enroll at any time during the year. To join a plan

141

you must be covered under both Medicare Part A and Part B and you must live in the plan's area of service.

Except in a Health Care Prepayment Plan or HCPP (described later) or if you are covered under the ESRD provisions, you may not be denied enrollment because of an existing medical condition or a disability. You may not join a managed care plan if you are a dialysis or kidney transplant patient. If, however, you develop permanent kidney failure while already enrolled in a plan, the plan must continue to cover you.

Pros and Cons of Managed Care

◤ Pluses

With a managed care plan, your medical costs are more predictable than under traditional fee-for-service plans. Also, many plans cover items such as preventive care, prescription drugs, inoculations, and eye exams, all of which Medicare excludes.

Another benefit is that there is often little or no paperwork involved. Filing claims under managed care is different than in traditional Medicare. In managed care, provided you are using network approved doctors and have followed procedures, there are no claims to file. You usually simply pay a nominal co-pay at the time services are rendered. If your plan allows you access to non-network doctors (called a Point of Service plan), you must follow the claim process required by the plan you are in for those services.

◤ Minuses

A managed care plan has its own group of health care providers, including hospitals, doctors, specialists, labs, and other outpatient medical services. The requirements of each plan are different, but in general you will obtain all your medical care within the plan's network of providers, or from someone you are referred to by the plan.

Some plans (e.g., HMOs) require you to choose a primary care physician who will decide whether or not to authorize you to see other medical providers. These physicians are sometimes referred to as "gatekeepers" because they control your access to other doctors and medical services. This is the most restrictive type of managed care plan and it means that your choice of primary care physician is very important because s/he has almost exclusive control of your medical care.

Other managed care plans allow you to use providers either inside or outside the network, without a gatekeeper physician. While these plans are clearly more user-friendly, they may cost more than traditional Medicare when you use services outside the network.

Because of these restrictions, you risk being unsatisfied with the doctors available within the plan's network. But this risk may be negligible for you. The rewards of extra benefits and ease of use may well outweigh any concerns you have in the matter.

To understand how flexible the plan is, it is important to understand clearly whether you can go outside the plan's network of providers and still obtain some reimbursement. Some plans allow for reimbursement of part of the cost and other plans do not reimburse you at all. This is an important distinction which is explained more fully in the following section.

Types of Managed Care Plans

There are three types of managed care plans currently available to Medicare beneficiaries: Risk Plans, Cost Plans and Health Care Prepayment (HCPP) Plans. All three may not be available in your area at this time. They are significantly different from one another.

Risk Plans

In a Risk Plan, the managed care organization assumes all risk for your health care. It provides all the services covered by Medicare Part A and Part B, usually with no deductibles and with nominal co-payments. Most Medicare managed care contracts are Risk Plans. HMOs are typical Risk Plans.

A Risk Plan generally requires you to get all your medical care within the plan's network of providers or by specific referral from the plan. If it provides additional benefits beyond those generally provided by Medicare (e.g., preventive care, eye care), those benefits can either be free, or you may have to pay an additional premium. The risk plan can require you to pay for the additional services as a condition of joining the plan.

Except when obtaining emergency or urgently needed medical care while you are temporarily outside your plan area, the plan will not (nor will Medicare) pay for any services obtained outside the plan network. Therefore, any non-emergency care you seek outside the network will be completely at your own expense.

Some risk plans now offer a Point of Service (POS) option for members. This option allows you to go outside the plan's network for medical services. The exact coverage offered by this option varies by plan, but it allows you more flexibility in your medical care and you will receive reimbursement for some of the costs you incur. The requirements for referrals, the amount actually reimbursed and the procedures to be followed all differ from plan to plan. If this option is available, the plan usually charges you an additional premium for it.

Cost Plans

Like Risk Plans, these plans offer all traditional Medicare benefits, usually without deductibles and co-payments. They provide more choices when it comes to medical providers, however. You are not locked into the plan's approved medical professionals. By staying within the plan's network for treatment, you have the benefit of paying only a co-pay for medical visits. If you go outside the network, you will have the usual fee-for-service Medicare coverage with its deductibles and co-insurance payments.

Unlike Risk Plans, Cost Plans may not offer you any "free" extra services. If the plan offers preventive care, dental care, or other care not ordinarily available from Medicare, you will be charged a premium for the additional services. The choice about signing up for these services is up to you. The plan cannot require you to do so as a condition of joining.

If you go outside the plan for treatment, the plan probably will not pay for the cost but Medicare will under its usual terms. In the latter case, you will be subject to the limitations of Medicare's coverage and responsible for all deductibles and co-insurance payments.

Health Care Prepayment Plans (HCPP)

These plans are similar to Cost Plans in design: they offer options as to choice of medical provider within a network of providers, and they allow you to go outside the network to obtain care. But there can be significantly less insurance coverage offered in these plans than in either a Risk or Cost Plan because HCPP plans do *not* have to match all of Medicare's coverage. They also do not have to provide open enrollment periods when people with pre-existing conditions can enroll.

Since HCPP plans are not comparable in coverage to either traditional Medicare or the other types of Medicare managed care, caution is advised when choosing this option. It may be the right option for you, but these plans can be much more limited in their coverage.

Switching Plans

Some people love managed care plans, others hate them. Once enrolled in a managed care plan, you may stay in it as long as it has a contract with Medicare. You may switch from one managed care plan to another in your area. And, you may return to traditional fee-for-service Medicare coverage at any time.

Enrollment in a new managed care plan simply requires signing up with the plan. You will be automatically removed from your former plan and transferred to the new plan.

If you wish to switch back to fee-for-service Medicare, you need to contact your Social Security (or Railroad Retirement Board) office. You will be re-enrolled in regular Medicare coverage on the first day of the next month after your request is received. If you re-enroll in regular Medicare Part A and Part B, you need to consider whether or not to obtain Medigap coverage.

Points to Consider

Managed care can offer many benefits and close a number of gaps in Medicare's coverage. The key is to know exactly what the plan allows, so before signing up, consider the following questions and see how managed care fits with your lifestyle.

- What type of plan is it (Risk, Cost or HCPP)?

- Do you travel frequently or live part of the year in a different location? If so, a managed care plan that restricts you to certain doctors may be a problem.

- Are you comfortable with the selection of doctors provided by the plan's network?

- How do you get medical care outside of the plan?

- What will the plan pay for if you go outside the network?

- How do you get reimbursed if you go outside the plan, i.e., what kind of paperwork is involved?

- How likely is it that you will want to get treatment outside the network?

- Does the plan pay for additional services such as preventive care, eye care, dental care, and prescription drugs? At what cost to you?

- Is there a wide variety of specialists in the network?

- Are the affiliated doctors and hospitals conveniently located?

- How long has the managed care organization been in business?

- How long has it had a Medicare contract?

- Can you easily change primary care physicians?

- Can you have the primary care physician of your choice within the network?

- Is it easy to get in touch with your primary care physician?

- What is the co-pay per visit?

- Are you responsible for any deductibles?

- What happens if you need or choose to get care outside the provider network?

- How do you get reimbursed for emergency care obtained outside the network? Outside the area?

- Are there limits on the length of hospital stays or skilled nursing facility stays?

- What, if any, kind of long-term care is available?

- Are there limits on any specific services, e.g., mental health care, physical therapy, or speech therapy?

- What types of services are available for home health care?

You will probably have other questions as well. Managed care organizations come in many variations. Research their benefits thoroughly before making a decision. And, if possible, check on their user-friendliness with other members who are already in the plan.

Choices, Choices

If you feel a managed care plan is your best option, compare coverage among several plans if possible. To help with this, use a worksheet similar to the one shown.

Managed Care Plan Worksheet

Item	Plan 1	Plan 2	Plan 3
Plan name			
A. M. Best rating (if applicable)			
Monthly premium			
Annual cost			
Type of plan (Risk, Cost, HCPP)			
Deductibles			
Co-insurance (co-pays)			
Number of hospital days covered			
Number of Skilled Nursing Facility days covered			
Point of Service option cost			
Home health care coverage			
Prescription drug coverage			
Preventive care coverage			
Is care available outside the plan's medical network?			
Patient's share of costs for non-network medical services			
Out-of-network emergency services available			
Length of time in business			
Nearness to primary care physician's office			
How does the appeals process work?			
Nearness to member hospital			
Freedom of choice for primary care physician?			
Ability to switch primary care physician			
Telephone availability of primary care physician			
Qualified specialists available within network			
Ambulance services			
Patient references			
Other:			
Other:			

Appealing a Claim

Claim appeals under managed care are handled differently than under traditional Medicare. As discussed in Chapter 7, traditional Medicare has a very specific appeals process. And with traditional Medicare, most appeals are decided in the patient's favor.

Not so under managed care. Each managed care plan sets its own rules with respect to appeals. If you have been denied care, you must first appeal the decision to the plan itself. And so far, the statistics show that most managed care appeals are found in favor of the plan, not the patient.

Disagreements over care decisions are arguably the most widely heard complaint about managed care plans. To address patient complaints, HCFA recently issued requirements that must be followed by all Medicare managed care plans. By law, your plan's member materials must clearly state what the appeal process is and how to use it.

As a managed care member, you (or your representative) have the right to challenge a decision with which you disagree. The initial phase of the process can take up to 60 days. However, if the situation is life threatening or otherwise time sensitive, you now have the right to request an expedited review. An expedited review takes 72 hours or less. The appeal process works in the following way:

▰ *Expedited Review Requests*

Patient Requests

■ You, or your representative, have the right to request an expedited review if you believe that your health, life or ability to maintain maximum function is in jeopardy. The expedited review process takes up to 72 hours.

■ This request may be oral or written. The plan is not required to grant a patient's request for expedited review, but it must notify you of its decision within the 72 hour period. If the plan does not grant the request for the review, it must automatically transfer the request to the standard 60-day appeal process.

Physician Requests

■ Your physician may request an expedited determination or s/he may add his or her support to your request. Once a physician supports the request and states that time is of the essence for medical reasons, the plan *must* grant the request for expedited review and render a decision on the request within 72 hours (or sooner if the medical situation dictates).

Hospitalized Patient Requests

■ If you are hospitalized and appealing a discharge determination, you have a choice. You can use the plan's expedited review process or you can use the Peer Review Organization (PRO) immediate review process. This process is the same as that offered traditional Medicare beneficiaries and is explained in detail in Chapter 7.

■ The PRO review process offers financial protection for the beneficiary while the review process proceeds. The plan's expedited request does not afford any financial protection to the beneficiary during the process.

Standard Requests

■ You, your representative, or your physician may file the request and the request must be filed in writing. You must follow the instructions in your membership materials.

■ This review can take up to 60 days to process and the plan must give you its decision in writing. If it denies your request, the plan must also tell you how to file an appeal of its decision.

■ If your appeal is denied at the end of 60 day process, you may file a written Request for Reconsideration and the plan has 60 more days to reach a decision. The plan must give you an opportunity to submit evidence in support of your request.

■ If at the end of 60 days, your request is denied, the request will be forwarded to HCFA for its review. HCFA will make the final determination.

The appeal process can be frustrating, but you have every right to insist that you are given clear, written instructions about the procedures to follow and a clear, written explanation of the reasons for the decision rendered by the plan. Contact your local HCFA office (see Appendix I) for assistance if you do not receive the information you need to file an appeal.

Frequently Asked Questions

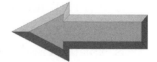

Q. How do managed care plans work?

A. Managed care plans have a network of health care professionals who offer coordinated medical services to enrolled plan members on a prepaid basis. Except in an emergency, services must be obtained from the medical providers and facilities that are part of the plan. If not, the member is liable for payment of all or part of the costs, depending upon the plan's rules. To use a medical service or professional outside the network, it is usually necessary to have your network doctor refer you to that provider.

Q. Can I use an HMO instead of a fee-for-service plan?

A. Yes. You may enroll in an HMO that has a contract with Medicare. Not all HMOs have contracts with Medicare, although more HMOs are approved by Medicare each year. To participate, you must live in the plan's service area and be enrolled in Medicare Part B.

HMO plans will provide all the Medicare-covered services; some plans also provide additional services for items such as vision care, dental care, and preventive care.

Q. What does it cost to join an HMO?

A. You will still pay the Medicare Part B monthly premium. The HMO may charge you an additional premium or a co-payment for services. The fees depend upon the services provided and the terms of the specific managed care plan.

Q. What is a Point of Service option?

A. Point of Service (POS) options allow you to go outside a plan's network of doctors. This optional coverage gives you more freedom of choice in getting medical care, but your plan will probably charge an additional premium for it. How much of the cost will be reimbursed and the procedure for going outside the network are determined by each plan.

Q. Are the co-pays and premiums regulated by Medicare?

A. No. The plans can set their own co-pay rates and premiums for extra services because different plans offer different services. The basic Part B premium which you pay each month is the only premium which is regulated by Medicare.

Q. If I enroll in a managed care plan, can I change my mind and go back to fee-for-service Medicare coverage?

A. Yes. You have the option to leave a managed care plan at any time. Just be careful to coordinate the start and end dates of your coverage since your coverage under fee-for-service Medicare does not begin until the first day of the month following your notification to Social Security that you want to switch. Make certain that your managed care plan coverage continues until your fee-for-service coverage begins again.

Q. I want to switch from one managed care program to another in my area. Is that possible?

A. Yes. You may switch from one plan to another Medicare approved plan simply by enrolling in the second plan. You will automatically be removed from the membership list of your prior plan.

Q. If my managed care plan is a cost plan, can I use doctors outside the network?

A. Yes. If the doctors are not part of the plan's list of providers, you will be covered by the regular Medicare benefits. You will be responsible for deductibles and co-insurance payments for these services the same as in a fee-for-service situation.

Q. If my plan is a Risk Plan, can I use doctors outside the network?

A. Yes, but you will be responsible for all the costs, as Medicare benefits will not apply.

Q. I was enrolled in an HMO at work and want to stay in that plan after retirement. Can I?

A. Only if the plan has a contract with Medicare to provide services.

Q. If I enroll in a managed care plan, will my access to a second opinion be restricted?

A. Possibly. In general, Medicare encourages and pays for second opinions. However, depending upon which type of managed care plan you are in, your primary care physician may be able to restrict your access to a second opinion because of the referral requirement.

Q. What is the difference between a managed care plan and an HMO?

A. An HMO is a type of managed care plan.

Q. Can I appeal the decision if my managed care plan won't pay for treatment?

A. Yes. You must file the appeal with your plan according to the instructions they give to you. The procedure for filing appeals should be in the member materials which the plan issues to you.

Q. Can someone else file an appeal for me?

A. You can designate someone to be your representative and s/he can file the appeal request, or your doctor can file the request.

Q. What kind of decisions can be appealed?

A. You can appeal managed care plan decisions about:

- refusing to pay a bill
- refusing to pay the full amount of a bill
- refusing to continue medical care that you believe is needed
- refusing to start medical care that you believe is needed

Q. What happens if I need a decision right away?

A. If the situation is health threatening and therefore you need a quick answer, you should file a request for expedited review. This process takes 72 hours. The plan does not have to grant the request, but it does have to respond to the request within the 72 hour time period.

Q. Is there any way to insist that the plan render a decision within 72 hours?

A. You can't "insist," but if your physician makes the request or supports your request, the plan must render the decision within 72 hours. The plan cannot ignore a physician's request for expedited review.

Q. Can I appeal if my plan denies my request for an expedited review?

A. No, but you can file a grievance with the plan. The plan must tell you how this procedure works.

Q. Is there any way to file a complaint about my plan if it doesn't follow the rules?

A. Yes. You can file a complaint about the quality of your care either with the plan itself or with the Peer Review Organization (PRO) in your area (see Appendix C). It may not change your situation, but it may help to have the problem corrected for the future.

CHAPTER **10**

Medicare Faces the Millenium

Medicare and the Balanced Budget Act of 1997

In 1997, Congress used the Balanced Budget Act of 1997 to substantively alter the Medicare program. The goal was to cut $115 billion dollars from Medicare's projected costs over the next five years.

Most of the changes were focused on cutting the payments made to the hospitals and other medical providers who treat Medicare patients. This type of change will be felt indirectly by patients as hospitals and medical providers deal with the new limitations.

The changes Congress made that affect Medicare beneficiaries directly include improved access to preventive screenings for breast cancer and colorectal cancer; improved diabetes self-management programs; slightly increased deductibles for 1998; the gradual shifting of home health care costs to Part B over the next six years; and a greater range of plan options beyond traditional Medicare.

In altering Medicare, Congress is following the blueprint laid out by corporate America in the last decade: encourage preventive care and shift the focus to managed care. All changes are aimed at lowering overall costs and slowing the spiraling cost of Medicare.

The new types of plans offer a variety of innovative ways to deliver Medicare coverage to beneficiaries. Two of the new plans are aimed specifically at Medicare recipients of substantial financial means, and the others are designed to make managed care more attractive to a larger number of beneficiaries. The down side for Medicare enrollees is that more choices probably means more confusion.

Health care providers will immediately feel the pinch of the new regulations. Lower payments will place all providers under more pressure to cut their own costs. Home health care agencies are also being scrutinized carefully to expose the filing of fraudulent claims. Whether revised payment limitations and reduction in payments to hospitals, doctors and other medical providers will affect the treatment and care of patients remains to be seen. Since cutting costs usually involves staffing cuts and service reductions, one can assume patients will feel some effect.

For people covered by traditional Medicare, out-of-pocket costs for deductibles and co-payments will go up slightly this year. A little publicized change has potentially costly ramifications. Some home health care services will move from Part A to Part B, subjecting these services to the Part B deductible and 20 percent co-payment. This shifting of home care coverage will be phased in over six years, so each year Part B coverage will cover more of the services needed for home care and be more of a necessity for those using home care services.

▰ The Particulars

The changes affecting beneficiaries are summarized as follows:

- Mammograms will be available annually, with no Part B deductible

- Pap smears and pelvic exams will be available every three years, with no Part B deductible

- Annual pap smears and pelvic exams for women at high risk of cervical or vaginal cancer, with no Part B deductible

- Annual screening for colorectal cancer using a fecal occult blood test for those aged 50 and over

- Screening colonoscopy for detection of colorectal cancer every 24 months for people at high risk

- Screening flexible sigmoidoscopy for detection of colorectal cancer every 48 months for those aged 50 and older

- Diabetes outpatient self-management training in ambulatory settings is added effective 7/1/98

- Blood glucose monitoring and testing strips are covered, effective 7/1/98

- Bone mass measurement testing to screen for osteoporosis is covered, effective 7/1/98

- No change in the Part B annual deductible or co-insurance percentage

- No change in the part B premium ($43.80 per month)

- Part A hospital deductible is increased to $764 per Benefit Period

■ Part A hospital co-insurance increased to $191 a day for days 61-90 and to $382 a day for each Lifetime Reserve Day

■ Skilled Nursing Facility co-insurance increased to $95.50 a day, days 21 –100 per Benefit Period

■ Switching of some home health care costs from Part A coverage to part B coverage (gradual implementation over 6 years)

■ Establishment of Part C, Medicare+Choice program for 1999

▰ How and When

The deductible and preventive care changes are effective in 1998. HCFA has until June 1998 to set up the formats and regulations for the plans which will be available under Medicare+Choice, and all these plans will be available by January 1, 1999.

HCFA must disseminate information about the new Medicare+Choice plans by November 1998, at which time beneficiaries will have the opportunity to choose which plan they wish to be covered by effective January 1, 1999. Traditional Medicare (Part A and Part B) will still be available as well.

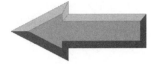

Frequently Asked Questions

Q. What are the 1998 deductibles?

A. The Part A hospital deductible is $764 per Benefit Period. For Part B, the deductible remains the same at $100 per year.

Q. What are the co-insurance payments for Part A and Part B?

A. For Part A:

- Days 61 – 90 in a hospital: $191 per day per Benefit Period

- Hospital Lifetime Reserve Days: $382 per day

- Days 21 – 100 in a Skilled Nursing Facility: $95.50 per day per Benefit Period

For Part B:

- Twenty percent (20%) co-insurance

Q. Do I have to use a managed care plan?

A. No. Traditional Part A and Part B Medicare will still be available. Choosing to use a managed care option under Medicare+Choice is completely optional.

Q. I am enrolled in a Medicare HMO now, what will happen to my coverage?

A. All existing Medicare managed care plans, including HMOs, will have to meet the new regulations under Medicare+ Choice regulations. Existing plans will have to be re-certified by HCFA to remain in the Medicare program. You will then be able to choose from among all the plans that are certified in your area.

Q. If I switch to a Medicare managed care plan, can I go back to regular Medicare?

A. Yes. For 1998, you may switch back at any time and your coverage will begin on the 1st day of the next month. Beginning in 2002, there will be restrictions on how often you can switch back and forth.

161

Q. What happens to my Medigap policy if I go into managed care?

A. You probably won't need it, depending upon the coverage given to you under the new plan. But, you may want to keep it until you are sure you are going to stay in the new plan because if you go back to Part A and Part B Medicare, you may be subject to pre-existing condition exclusions on the Medigap policy. So just be sure you don't need it before you cancel it.

Q. What is Medicare Part C?

A. Medicare Part C contains all the non-traditional and managed care Medicare plans. It is also known as Medicare+ Choice (see Chapter 11).

Q. When do I have to decide about Medicare+Choice plans?

A. HCFA will should notify you about the options available in your area in November 1998. You will then be able to make a choice among the available plans, which will be effective January 1, 1999.

Medicare+Choice

Medicare +Choice

The Medicare+Choice (Part C) program will include all of the optional plan designs other than traditional Medicare which are available under the new regulations. The options that will be available beginning January 1, 1999 run the gamut from new and expanded managed care plans to innovative insurance plans which are targeted at higher income Medicare beneficiaries.

The choices offered will give a wider array of options to beneficiaries and offer more flexibility in managed care options. The plans will also be available in all regions of the country.

When deciding whether to opt for one of the new plans, it is important to review all the plans available in your area and compare them to the benefits available under traditional Medicare. The final decision will be based on individual factors such as finances, health status and plan coverage. There are some interesting alternatives being proposed, but they may or may not fit your particular situation.

To encourage people to try the new plans, Medicare will allow you to switch back to traditional Medicare at any time without penalty. (Although there could be some pre-existing illness issues with your Medigap policy, so exercise caution.)

Until 2002, Medicare+Choice enrollees may switch back to traditional Medicare at any time and the change will be effective with the next month. (Beginning in 2002, there will be limitations on the number of times and periods when such switches may be made.)

It is more important than ever to be an educated Medicare consumer when making your plan decision. Fortunately, at this time it is not an irrevocable decision.

◤ When Is a Government Program Not Exactly a Government Program?

In traditional Medicare Part A and Part B, your coverage is provided by the government through HCFA. You deal with Medicare through approved Medicare Carriers and Intermediaries who may or may not be insurance companies. These Carriers and Intermediaries are simply agents for HCFA who process Medicare claims for them and are paid a fee for rendering this service. They handle the paperwork, but the government insures you and assumes all the risks associated with paying your claims.

This is not the case with Part C plans. While the funding for medical care still comes through HCFA, Part C plans are not run by HCFA. They are regulated by HCFA and overseen by HCFA, but they are independent entities.

This is an important difference because it affects your benefits, the claims process and the appeals process. Part C plans are individual plans which can be established by insurance companies, non-profit organizations, groups of health care providers or others who meet the regulations.

The coverage provided to you as a plan member must meet minimum standards established by HCFA for that type of plan, but each organization has the ability to alter this coverage by adding other coverage, by charging for plan options, by restricting your use of medical providers, or by otherwise "customizing" their particular plan.

Because of this, it is important to carefully compare the plans which are offered in your area. Beyond the basics required by HCFA, each plan has features which are specific to it. These items should be made clear in the literature provided to you by the plan. To address its concern about the possibility of misleading information being disseminated, all marketing materials which are used by these plans must be approved in advance by HCFA. Hopefully, this will make the documents accurate, but they still may not be completely clear so ask all the questions you need to before making a decision.

▰ Just When You Thought You Understood Medicare — More Choices

Part C is an alphabet soup of choices. There are managed care plans (or as Medicare prefers to call them, coordinated care plans), catastrophic care plans, religious and fraternal plans, and even a Private Fee-for-Service plan. It seems HCFA is trying to develop something for everyone and to provide plan options that suit a wide array of personal situations.

To be eligible for a Medicare+Choice plan, you must be enrolled in both Medicare Part A and Part B. You will continue to pay the Part B monthly premium after you are enrolled in a Medicare+Choice.

The plan options to be included in Medicare+Choice are:

- Health Maintenance Organizations (HMOs)
- Preferred Provider Organizations (PPOs)
- Preferred Sponsor Organizations (PSOs)
- Medical Savings Accounts (MSAs)
- *Private* Fee-for-Service Plans (PFFS)
- Religious and Fraternal Plans

The Medicare +Choice Plans

▰ *Coordinated Care or Managed Care Plans*

These plans will play a major role in the Part C coverage and they have certain common characteristics.

- They have a network of doctors, hospitals and other medical providers which are preferred by the plan. There are financial incentives to use these providers and it will cost you more to go outside of the network, although the specifics of these financial consequences vary by plan.

- They generally require you to choose a Primary Care physician who will coordinate all your medical care. Some plans require the approval of this Primary Care Physician before you may obtain care from another medical professional (either in or out of the network). While other plans allow you a certain freedom of choice with respect to your doctors.

- They may offer preventive and other medical services which are not covered by traditional Medicare. Depending upon the plan chosen, these services

(e.g., preventive care, eye care, and dental care)
may be included free of charge to you or they may
be purchased at an additional premium.

■ They do not cover hospice care.

■ You usually do not need to have a Medigap policy.

■ They are available in specific geographic areas.

There will be three types of coordinated care plans available
under Medicare+Choice:

1. **Health Maintenance Organizations (HMO)** — This is the most
   restrictive type of managed care plan. All patient care is
   directed by one primary care or gatekeeper physician
   and plan members must use the medical providers who
   are part of the plan's network.

   The primary care physician controls access to specialists
   and other medical services. Provided s/he authorizes the
   care, the costs are covered. There may be a small co-pay
   due at the time medical services are rendered. Services
   rendered outside the network are not usually reimburs-
   able to the patient.

2. **Preferred Provider Organizations (PPO)** — These plans are
   composed of a group of doctors, hospitals and other
   medical providers from whom enrollees may obtain
   treatment. There may be a primary care physician,
   but this doctor does not control access to medical
   services in the same restrictive way that a gatekeeper
   physician in an HMO can.

   A patient can get care from a provider within the group
   or from outside the group. There is a financial incentive

for the patient to obtain care within the PPO's network because there is usually a smaller out-of-pocket cost if s/he stays within the group. This amount varies depending on the particular plan and the services included, but within the plan the patient usually pays only a nominal co-pay at the time of service. By going outside the plan's provider list, the patient is usually responsible for a much higher co-insurance payment and, possibly, a deductible.

3. **Provider Sponsored Organizations (PSO)** — This is a completely new addition to the Medicare coordinated care mix. It is a public or private entity established by health care providers, which provides a substantial portion of health care services directly or through affiliated providers. The providers and affiliates share the financial risk of providing these services.

▰ Catastrophic Care Plan

Medical Savings Accounts (MSA) — These plans combine a high deductible (catastrophic) health insurance policy with a tax-advantaged savings account. Medicare would pay for the cost of the catastrophic care insurance policy and any remaining balance would be deposited in the beneficiary's MSA account.

The money in the account accumulates tax-free and may be used to pay for the beneficiary's medical services, including services not usually covered by Medicare (e.g., eye care, dental care, mileage reimbursement for medical care). Once the $6000 deductible is met, the insurance policy would pay for all Medicare covered services. The MSA program will have a limited enrollment.

◤ *Other Plans*

Private Fee-for-Service Plans — These plans set their own fee schedule for hospital, doctor and other medical provider care. Beneficiaries may see any provider who agrees to the plan's fee schedule. These plans are aimed at wealthier Medicare enrollees and are not subject to Medicare's limitations on fees or its fee schedule.

Religious and Fraternal Benefit Society Plans — These plans may restrict enrollment to Medicare beneficiaries who are members of the religious group or fraternal organization. The plan design and benefits would be up to the sponsoring group.

Enrolling in Part C (Medicare +Choice) Eligibility requirements for Part C plans are the same as for Medicare Part A and Part B. To participate in a Part C plan, you will have to be enrolled in both Part A and Part B and you will continue to be charged the Part B premium monthly.

All Medicare Part C plans will be available beginning January 1, 1999. In November 1998, HCFA will publicize the specifics of the Medicare+Choice plans that are available in each region and you will be able to enroll in the plan of your choice. You may choose to remain with traditional Medicare coverage, and if you do not choose, you will be placed in the traditional program.

This November enrollment period will be repeated annually so that beneficiaries may choose the plan they wish to have for the following calendar year. Initially, you will be able to switch back to traditional Medicare coverage at any time if you are dissatisfied with your Part C plan.

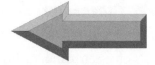

Frequently Asked Questions

Q. What is the difference between Medicare managed care and Medicare+Choice?

A. Medicare+Choice includes several types of non-traditional insurance plans. Among these are several managed care plans.

Q. What is Part C?

A. It is the Medicare+Choice program and it includes all of the non-traditional Medicare plans.

Q. What is a Medical Savings Account?

A. Medical Savings Accounts (MSAs) combine high deductible ($6000) health coverage with a tax advantaged savings plan. The funds in the savings account may be used to pay for medical expenses, even those which are not usually covered by Medicare.

Q. What is Private Fee-for-Service plan?

A. This is a plan which will set its own fee schedule with doctors, hospitals and other medical service providers. Subscribers to this plan will be able to see any provider who agrees to this private fee schedule. The plan is designed for people of substantial financial means, as Medicare's limitations on fees will not apply.

Q. When can I sign up for a Medicare+Choice plan?

A. The initial enrollment period will begin in November for plans available January 1, 1999.

Q. **What can I do if I don't like the Part C plan after I enroll?**

A. You may leave that plan and switch back to traditional Medicare at any time. Your traditional Medicare will be back in force on the 1st of the next month.

Q. **I'm already in a Medicare HMO. What will happen to my coverage?**

A. In November, you will have to choose from among the Medicare+Choice plans that are offered in your area. If your existing plan is still available, you can stay in it. If it isn't available, you will have to choose a different plan.

Q. **Do I need a Medigap policy with the managed care options in Part C?**

A. You don't need the Medigap policy as it probably duplicates your coverage in the managed care plan.

Q. **Why would I keep my Medigap policy after I join a Medicare+Choice managed care plan?**

A. Until you are certain that you are going to stay in the Medicare+Choice plan, it is prudent not to cancel your Medigap policy. You don't need it to supplement the managed care coverage, but it protects you from a pre-existing illness exclusion if you decide to switch back to Part A and Part B coverage.

Q. **If I go from Medicare+Choice to traditional Medicare, will I have a problem with pre-existing condition exclusions?**

A. You should be okay with respect to your Medicare coverage, but your Medigap coverage could have an exclusion if you have cancelled it. Check with your Medigap insurer to be sure.

SECTION IV
OTHER CONSIDERATIONS

CHAPTER **12**

Medicaid

How Medicaid Works

The services and medical care provided under a state's Medicaid program can be provided separately from Medicare, or in some instances, in conjunction with Medicare.

Eligibility for Medicaid assistance is based solely on financial need. The largest portion of Medicaid funds are spent on the elderly, but Medicaid also covers numerous people, including children, who are not eligible for Medicare.

Medicaid programs are run by the states, with the benefits provided and the requirements for eligibility determined on a state by state basis. The state gets a portion of the funding for its Medicaid program from the federal government, so the coverage provided is based on guidelines issued at the federal level. But each state works out its own program within the guidelines. And with the new push in Washington to lower the cost of Medicaid, the states are being given ever more flexibility in deciding how to spend the money.

For many elderly Medicare recipients, Medicaid assistance becomes a necessity. This occurs because of the financial problems caused by payments for long-term nursing home care or for high medical bills from a catastrophic illness. Since Medicare does not cover custodial care and most nursing home stays exceed 30 months in length, many Medicare beneficiaries exhaust their financial resources long before their need for care ends. The costs associated with an extended nursing home stay or the expenses associated with catastrophic illnesses can overwhelm personal savings very quickly.

One chapter cannot cover all the ins and outs of Medicaid. Rather, this chapter explains the basic issues surrounding how Medicaid can affect people who also qualify for Medicare coverage. Assistance for medical care under the Medicaid program can be provided for people who are currently Medicare eligible and also for people who receive Supplementary Security Income (SSI) benefits from Social Security.

Depending upon your financial situation and medical needs, Medicaid may help in several ways. For information on any of these programs, contact your state's Medicaid office (listed in Appendix E).

▼ Qualified Medicare Beneficiaries (QMB)

This program will pay for a person's Medicare Part B premium. Usually it will also cover the Medicare Part A and Part B deductibles and co-payments.

To qualify:

- You must be eligible for Medicare Part A insurance.

- Your income must be below the federal poverty level.

- Your assets may not exceed $4000 for an individual or $6000 for a couple, although slightly higher amounts are allowable in Hawaii and Alaska.

▰ *Specified Low-Income Medicare Beneficiary (SLMB)*

People participating in this program are eligible for payment of their Medicare Part B premiums only. To qualify:

- You must be eligible for Medicare Part A coverage

- Your income must not exceed the national poverty level by more than 20 percent (slightly higher in Alaska and Hawaii).

▰ *Covered Expenses with Medicaid*

There are certain types of coverage which most states provide to Medicaid recipients, but—as with the financial requirements—each state has flexibility as to what services will be covered. For Medicare beneficiaries who are eligible for their state's Medicaid program, Medicaid will function as the secondary insurer.

The general types of coverage which may be provided, depending upon the state, include:

- Doctors and surgeons, inpatient or outpatient
- Dentists, podiatrists, psychologists, and optometrists
- Prescriptions
- Rural health clinic services
- Hospital care, inpatient and outpatient
- HMOs (in certain areas)
- Mental health services
- Medical supplies and equipment
- Prostheses, hearing aids, eyeglasses, and braces
- X-rays and lab services
- Hospice care

- Transportation to services, subject to certain limitations
- Personal care assistance
- Long-term care

Medicaid Eligibility

Eligibility for Medicaid is determined by state requirements in three areas:

- Proof of disability or age
- Income limitations
- Asset limitations

In brief, you have to show financial need, based on your state's formula for calculating the maximum allowable income and assets. This calculation excludes certain asset items and it varies depending upon the need for living expenses of a spouse, if any. Under no circumstances does it allow you to keep much in the way of a financial cushion.

To apply, you will have to disclose all assets and sources of income, and you may have to sell or turn over your ownership of some assets to the state in order to qualify. The formulas used and the types of assets which are counted are complicated. Should you exhaust your Medicare benefits and still require care, Medicaid is the place you will most likely look for assistance with medical bills, so it is advisable to learn about your state's requirements before you need the assistance. This is especially important for married couples, as the spouse who does not require long-term or catastrophic care can be left in a very uncertain financial situation.

If you are over 65, have an income (from all sources) below the state limitation, and do not have qualifying assets which exceed the state's requirements, you can qualify for assistance.

If your assets are above the allowable limits, you will have to nearly exhaust them before becoming eligible. This is referred to as "spending down." The limits and the types of income and assets counted also vary depending upon whether you have a spouse who requires support.

To obtain more information on Medicaid requirements in your state, check with the state's Medicaid office. These are listed in Appendix E of this book.

Medicare and Medicaid Coordination

A person may be eligible for both Medicare and Medicaid coverage. In this situation, your Medicare coverage will be primary with all available benefits being used before Medicaid kicks in. Medicaid may also pay for items which Medicare does not cover, but it is based on showing financial need and the state is rigorous in its search for assets and income.

If you are currently receiving Supplemental Security Income (SSI) payments from Social Security you are eligible for Medicaid. You must apply for it by contacting your state Medicaid office.

Frequently Asked Questions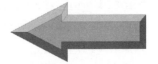

Q. I can't afford to pay for Medicare part B coverage. Is there anything I can do?

A. Yes. If your annual income is near the national poverty level and you do not have access to many financial resources, you may qualify for government assistance under your state's Medicaid program. The Qualified Medicare Beneficiary

(QMB) and the Specified Low-Income Medicare Beneficiary (SLMB) programs are designed to help pay Medicare's monthly premiums. The QMB program may also pay for some of the deductibles and co-insurance amounts. If you think you may qualify, you should contact your state or local welfare, social service, or public health agency.

Q. If I exhaust my financial resources because of medical bills that are not covered by Medicare, can I qualify for Medicaid assistance?

A. Yes. Qualifying for financial assistance depends upon the rules in your particular state. If you meet the income and asset tests in your state, you should seek assistance from the state Medicaid office.

Q. If my father is in a nursing home, will Medicaid pay for it?

A. If his income and assets meet the financial tests, most states will pay for nursing home care. This is one of Medicaid's largest expenditures.

Q. Is there any protection for my spouse if my assets are all spent on my medical bills?

A. There are federal guidelines which allow a person to qualify for Medicaid assistance without leaving a spouse penniless. Certain assets can be retained and some level of income, but it isn't a lot. The chances are that your spouse will be in a precarious financial position.

Q. What is "spending down"?

A. If a person has more assets and income than is allowable to qualify for Medicaid, s/he can deplete his/her assets to meet the income and asset levels. For example, if someone is in a nursing home, s/he will first have to spend his/her financial resources on the costs for staying there. Once these resources have been depleted sufficiently, the person can qualify for Medicaid. The process of using up available income and assets is called "spending down."

Q. Can I just transfer my assets to my children and then apply for Medicaid?

A. No. There are many restrictions on such transfers and there are minimum time limits that must pass before the transferred funds are actually unavailable for Medicaid purposes. If you are thinking of transferring assets, consult an attorney.

Q. Where do I get information on Medicaid?

A. Contact your state's Medicaid office. These are listed in Appendix E.

Q. What if I just don't tell the state about all my assets?

A. This is fraud and is subject to criminal penalties. The Medicaid authorities are pretty adept at finding assets, so this is not the solution.

Q. Is there any way to protect my assets from being counted?

A. Yes. Assets may be transferred and/or placed in certain types of trusts. There are strictly enforced rules as to when assets must have been transferred or put in trust. This is a complex subject and you should seek advice from a professional who is knowledgeable about trusts and elder law.

CHAPTER 13

Medicare and Other Medical Insurance

Coordination of Benefits

Some people eligible for Medicare also have access to medical insurance coverage from other sources. In these cases, the other coverage will affect how Medicare pays for services and the options for enrolling in Medicare.

The most common situation is that of a person over 65 who is working for a company that provides health insurance coverage for its employees. Under federal law, companies with 20 employees or more must provide the same coverage to employees over 65 as to anyone else in the health care plan. The group's health plan may have many of the same or better benefits than Medicare would offer.

If a person has employer-provided group health coverage, the company's insurance carrier is the primary payer of medical expenses and Medicare becomes the secondary payer. All medical bills must be submitted to the company's insurer first. If any charges remain unpaid, they are sent to Medicare for reimbursement.

This combination can cause confusion and billing errors by medical providers. It is a relatively uncommon situation and many providers simply assume that Medicare is primary, even if they have been told otherwise. If the bills are submitted to Medicare first, they will be rejected, causing delays in payment and unnecessary paperwork headaches. If you are in this situation, bring it to the attention of the person requesting your insurance information.

If you are covered under an employer-sponsored group plan, you may decide not to accept Medicare Part B coverage. (Since Medicare Part A is free for qualified beneficiaries there is little reason not to sign up for it.) If you do not participate in Part B while in the group's health plan, you have the option of enrolling within eight months of the termination of either the coverage or your employment. This "special enrollment period" only applies to people with group coverage. It means that they do not need to wait for a general enrollment period in order to apply for Medicare. There is also no penalty added to the Medicare Part B premium for the delay in enrollment.

It is possible that you or your spouse may have private insurance that can be continued after age 65. Before making any decisions about your Medicare coverage you should review your policy carefully to make certain that your benefits remain the same after age 65. Unlike group medical coverage, some private policies change coverage after age 65 on the assumption that the policyholder will be eligible for Medicare.

Whatever the case, never cancel any insurance until you have confirmation that your Medicare coverage is in effect.

Group Plans vs. Medicare

It is quite possible that the coverage available to you under a group plan will be as good as or better than your Medicare coverage. Should you decide against getting Medicare Part B, it is strongly recommended that you sign up for Part A Medicare if you are eligible. It won't cost anything and it is additional coverage.

To help decide the question, use a worksheet similar to the one that follows to compare your options.

Group Health Insurance Worksheet

Item	Medicare Part A	Medicare Part A & B	Medicare & Medigap	Group Policy
Monthly Cost				
Deductibles				
Co-insurance				
Annual/Lifetime Benefit Limits				
Annual out-of-pocket limits				
Pre-existing condition limitations				
Preventive care				
Prescriptions				
Long-term care				
Hospital days covered				
Skilled Nursing Facility days covered				
Home health care services				
Managed care plan				
Other:				

183

Frequently Asked Questions

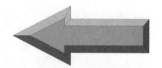

Q. Is Medicare always the primary payer of a beneficiary's medical bills?

A. No. There are a number of situations in which another insurer is the primary payer of your health care costs and Medicare is the secondary payer. For example, Medicare may be the secondary payer if you are covered by an employer's group health insurance plan, or are entitled to veterans benefits, workers' compensation, or black lung benefits. Medicare also may be the secondary payer if no-fault insurance or liability insurance (such as automobile insurance) is available as the primary payer.

In cases where Medicare is the secondary payer, Medicare may pay some or all of the charges not paid by the primary payer for services and supplies covered by Medicare.

Q. I am over 65 and have full group health benefits at my job; do I need Medicare?

A. If your group coverage pays for the same or better benefits than Medicare, you probably don't need both. But the only way to know is to compare both plans carefully and compare the cost to you for the coverage. You should consider getting Part A coverage anyway, even if you don't get Part B. Part A is free to eligible beneficiaries and it will be secondary to your group health insurance.

Q. I am 70 and have group health coverage from my employer. When I retire and my coverage ceases, can I get Medicare?

A. Yes. Apply for Medicare and be sure to explain that you are now covered by a group policy. You may pay a penalty if you aren't already signed up for Part A coverage, but you won't pay a penalty on the Part B coverage. You also won't have to wait for the annual enrollment periods to sign up; there is a special enrollment period in this case.

Q. My health insurance paid some of my claims for a recent illness. I have both Part A and Part B. Will Medicare pay the difference?

A. Submit the claims and, if they are approved Medicare costs, Medicare will pay its share.

Q. I know my health insurance doesn't pay for certain types of costs that Medicare does. Do I always have to submit my claim to them first?

A. Yes. Medicare will simply reject the claim unless it sees proof (the other claim notification will do) that the primary insurance company has not paid for it.

Q. My employer's group coverage is with an HMO. Does this mean I can't also have Medicare?

A. No. If you are eligible for Medicare, you can sign up for it if you want it.

Q. If my employer's group coverage is an HMO, do I have to use a Medicare HMO for my other coverage?

A. No. You can choose whatever type of Medicare coverage makes sense for you. Medicare will simply be secondary to your employer's HMO coverage.

Q. I can continue with my employer's plan after I retire. Why get Medicare?

A. Check with your employer and make sure that your coverage doesn't change after retirement. Unless your group has 20 or more people in it, the group plan may only offer Medigap coverage to retirees. If that is the case, you will need to have Medicare coverage as well.

CHAPTER **14**

Your Financial Exposure

**Medicare &
Personal
Finances**

Now that you have a handle on what
Medicare does pay for, let's focus on what
is missing. The gaps in Medicare's coverage
leave people vulnerable to medical expenses
that can seriously undermine their financial
security. Unanticipated and uninsured medical expenses can
mount quickly, as we all know. This affects the patient, the
patient's spouse, and the patient's family.

Insufficient insurance coverage can have many consequences,
among them:

- Lack of insurance can undermine someone's ability
  to obtain desired medical assistance.

- Expenditures for uninsured medical treatment can
  rapidly deplete a patient's financial resources and
  jeopardize his/her ability to handle other living
  expenses.

- The cost of medical treatment may create a financial strain for other family members if they have to
  supplement the insurance payments for needed
  treatment.

186

■ Depleting financial resources can leave a surviving spouse or life partner in a precarious financial state or compromise his/her independence because of a need to rely upon the generosity of other family members.

■ Lack of insurance coverage and/or funds for home-based assistance or for long-term care may force a family member to take on the full-time job of caretaker. This can cause loss of income and have a negative effect on the family member's other responsibilities.

There are many variations of the themes noted above. With a bit of thought, most people can probably come up with several examples in their own or their friend's families where a medical problem had a negative effect on someone's life and finances. The consequences of insufficient medical coverage are, at base, financial. But the lifestyle changes and life upheavals that can be caused along with the financial difficulties can be shattering to all involved.

Risk Management
Risk management is a term often heard in corporate settings, but it has relevance to personal situations as well. In essence, the term means that risk (in this case the potential for incurring large medical expenses) can be managed by careful evaluation of the options available.

Note that the term is not risk elimination. The total elimination of financial risk is not possible because a person cannot insure against every eventuality. And even if that were possible, the cost would be so prohibitive that very few people could afford such insurance.

For Medicare recipients, managing risk involves making an informed decision about how comfortable an individual is with the possibility of incurring large, non-reimbursed medical expenses. Not everyone has high medical costs and not everyone needs long-term care. The problem is, no one can tell if they will or will not have medical difficulties. And, in the case of married couples, two people are at risk for incurring large bills. Unfortunately, there isn't a perfect way to predict the eventuality of high medical expenses and the cost of trying to cover all the bases can be expensive in its own right.

How much risk to assume is a highly personal decision that can be made only by the person or persons involved. Many variables will enter into such a decision, including a person's current health, family medical history, financial situation, income level, availability of long-term care from family members or friends, etc.

It is not an easy call by any means, but the best way to decide is to evaluate the options available to reduce identifiable risks. To help, we will highlight the gaps in Medicare and discuss the available ways to plug those gaps.

Medicare's Gaps

As discussed in an earlier chapter, Medicare is a good, but not a perfect, system of health insurance. We will be illustrating the financial implications through the use of examples later, but first let's review the basic gaps in Medicare's coverage:

Part A does not pay:

- The deductible for the first admission to a hospital in any one Benefit Period. In 1998, the deductible is $764.

- The daily hospital co-insurance for inpatient hospital days 61 through 90 ($191 per day in 1998).

- Any charges incurred after 90 days in the hospital, unless the patient has some or all of his/her lifetime reserve days available. (There are 60 total lifetime reserve days available.)

- The daily co-insurance for each lifetime reserve day used ($382 per day in 1998).

- The cost of the first three pints of blood used, unless replaced.

- For a private room, unless medically necessary.

- For private duty nursing.

- For care in a hospital that is not part of the Medicare program, unless it is for emergency care.

- For care received outside the United States, except for certain limited circumstances in Mexico or Canada.

- For any care in a psychiatric hospital after using 190 days of such care in a lifetime.

- Daily co-insurance for days 21 through 100 in a skilled nursing facility in any one Benefit Period ($95.50 per day in 1998).

- For any costs in a skilled nursing facility after the 100th day in a Benefit Period.

- Any costs for a stay in a skilled nursing facility that are for custodial care, rather than for rehabilitation or other approved, medically necessary treatment.

- Physician or specialist expenses (such as for surgeons and anesthesiologists).

- Any costs for nursing home care or other care that is custodial in nature.

- Any costs for care in a skilled nursing facility if the patient is not transferred there within a timely manner after a qualifying stay in a hospital.

- For any costs in a skilled nursing facility that are not approved by Medicare.

- For full-time nursing care at home.

- For prescriptions, except those received during a qualifying hospital or skilled nursing facility stay.

- For in-home caretaker services that are designed to assist with personal living needs.

- The 20 percent co-insurance on the Medicare approved cost for durable medical equipment, or for any excess over the approved amount.

- The co-payments for outpatient drugs received under the hospice care program (five percent of the reasonable cost, not to exceed $5 per prescription).

Part B does not pay:

- Any of the costs listed under Part A above, except Medicare approved physician and specialist expenses.

- The annual deductible ($100 per year in 1998).

- The 20 percent co-payment on Medicare approved expenses (e.g., doctors' bills).

- Any charges above the Medicare approved amount for medical services or goods.

- Fifty percent of the Medicare approved amount for outpatient mental health services.

- For preventive care, except for mammograms, Pap smears, prostate cancer screening, and certain inoculations (flu, pneumonia, and Hepatitis B shots).

- For acupuncture, naturopathy, or other non-traditional forms of treatment.

- For dental expenses.

- For eye examinations or expenses, except for prosthetic lenses required after cataract surgery.

- For hearing examinations or hearing aids.

- For podiatry or other foot care services, unless related to a covered condition such as diabetes.

- Any charges incurred outside the United States, except in limited situations for care in Mexican or Canadian hospitals.

- Charges for the first three pints of blood annually, unless replaced or the three-unit deductible is met during a hospital stay.

This is a pretty long list when you look at the missing pieces. And, without Part B coverage, the gaps are even more substantial. Clearly, Medicare pays for numerous items, but just as clearly each person needs to understand exactly what it doesn't cover in order to protect himself/herself financially.

191

Benefit Periods and the Medicare Calendar

Before proceeding to hypothetical situations with dollars, let's review how Benefit Periods work and how they affect deductibles and co-payments. Different types of services are subject to different limitations. Part A Benefit Periods can have a substantial effect on the amount of money that a patient can be out of pocket with Medicare.

Medicare Part A pays hospital expenses and skilled nursing facility expenses based on Benefit Periods. The Benefit Period starts with the hospital admission and continues until the patient has been out of the hospital or skilled nursing facility for a period of 60 days. Part A expenses for home health care and hospice care are not subject to this Benefit Period restriction.

Medicare Part B expenses are calculated on an annual basis, so the calendar year is the Benefit Period for these medical costs.

Let's look at the easier Part B Benefit Period first, as most people are familiar with looking at medical and other expenses on an annual calendar year basis:

▰ Part B Examples

1. Ann has high blood pressure and visits her doctor every three months for a checkup and a review of her medication. In this calendar year, she has had three appointments so far at a cost of $75 each ($225 total) and has not had any other Medicare covered medical expenses.

    These expenses will be covered under her Part B coverage and therefore the Benefit Period is the calendar year. Ann met her $100 deductible as a result of the cost of her first two appointments. It does not matter how many more times she goes to the doctor or how long the time period is between visits, this $100 is the only deductible she will be subject to in this calendar year (for Medicare Part B expenses).

2. In addition to the physician she consults about her blood pressure, Ann also is treated by another physician for her asthma. She will have one appointment later in the calendar year. Since she has already met her $100 annual deductible by her visits to the doctor listed in example 1, she is not subject to paying the deductible again. She is still in the same calendar year Benefit Period.

Less easily understood are Benefit Periods as defined in Medicare Part A coverage.

▰ Part A Examples

1. Sally fell and broke her hip six months ago. She was admitted to the hospital and remained there for 21 days, at which point she was discharged. She went home and has not been readmitted to the hospital for any reason. Her Benefit Period began the day she was admitted, she used up 21 days of hospital coverage in the Benefit Period, and she did not reenter the hospital within 60 days of discharge. Should she ever have to be readmitted, she will start a new Benefit Period.

2. John fell and injured his back. He was admitted to the hospital for surgery and remained there for 21 days. He was discharged and transferred immediately to a skilled nursing facility for rehabilitation. He was in the rehabilitation facility for 28 days, and then discharged. After three weeks at home, he was readmitted to the hospital for further treatment due to complications. The new hospitalization was day 50 (21 hospital days + 28 skilled nursing facility days =

49 benefit days used) of his original Benefit Period because he returned to the hospital within 60 days of his discharge from the rehabilitation facility.

3. Patty suffered a stroke and was hospitalized for 18 days, after which she was transferred to a rehabilitation center. She stayed in this skilled nursing facility for 38 days, then was admitted to an intermediate care facility since she still needed some help caring for herself and also was receiving some therapy. She required assistance with dressing, personal hygiene, getting in and out of bed, eating and other daily activities. After one month, she suffered another stroke, was readmitted to the hospital, and treated for 14 days. She was then released and returned to the intermediate care facility.

The initial hospitalization and rehab used up 56 days (18+38) in her Benefit Period. Since she was readmitted to the hospital within 60 days of discharge from the skilled nursing facility, her second hospitalization started on the 57th day of the Benefit Period and ended on the 71st day of the original Benefit Period. She received Medicare benefits for the days spent in the hospital and rehabilitation center, but there was no coverage for the time spent in the intermediate care facility.

The Arithmetic of Medicare

The best way to view the financial impact of the gaps in Medicare's coverage is to look at a few examples. All examples assume the patient has both Part A and Part B coverage.

1. Tom was hospitalized for 14 days during which time he had hip surgery, and his doctor visited him once per day.

He was discharged from the hospital to a skilled nursing facility where he stayed for nine days before transferring to an intermediate care facility for one month.

Medicare pays for everything, except:

- Hospital Part A deductible: $764 $ 764.00

- Part B deductible: $100   100.00

- Co-pay on 14 doctor visits:
  20% of $600 (14 visits at $50 per visit,
  minus $100 deductible)   120.00

- Co-pay on surgeon's bill:
  20% of $4500   900.00

- All costs at intermediate care facility:
  30 days at $125 per day   3,750.00

  Total out-of-pocket costs $5,634.00

2. Jane went to her internist four times a year for checkups because of her high blood pressure and diabetes. Each doctor's visit was $75 and her prescriptions cost $180 per month.

   Medicare paid for everything except:

   - Annual Part B deductible: $100 $ 100.00

   - Co-pay on doctor visits:
     20% of $200 (4 visits at $75 per visit,
     minus $100 deductible)   40.00

   - Prescriptions: 12 months at $180   2,160.00

     Total out-of-pocket costs $2,300.00

3.   Larry had a severe stroke. He was hospitalized for 22 days, and his doctor visited him daily at $50 per visit. He was discharged to a skilled nursing facility. He stayed at the skilled nursing facility for 54 days receiving rehabilitation. He was then moved to a nursing home because he was unable to care for himself at home; he remained there for 12 months. While in the nursing home he received physical therapy three times per week at $75 per session and his prescriptions cost $425 per month.

Medicare paid for everything except:

- Hospital deductible: $764 $ 764.00

- Annual Part B deductible   100.00

- Co-pay on doctor visits:
  20% of $1,000 (22 visits at $50 per visit,
  minus $100 deductible)   200.00

- Daily co-pay for 34 days at SNF
  at $95.50 (Days 21–54)   3,247.00

- Nursing home care: 365 days at $125   45,625.00

- Co-pay on physical therapy at
  nursing home: 20% of $11,700
  (52 weeks × 3 sessions at $75)   2,340.00

- Prescription costs: 12 months
  at $425 per month   5,100.00

  Total out-of-pocket costs $57,376.00

These examples illustrate how quickly costs can mount. When looking at a chart of Medicare deductibles and co-payments, none seem terribly high. But when added together in a real life medical situation, those numbers can be staggering. The examples above include basic types of medical care. In a real hospitalization, there will be more doctors and more specialists, so these hospitalization examples are probably low for the situations described. And the typical nursing home resident is there for 30 months.

In summary, your financial exposure is fairly large due to Medicare's gaps and you need to take precautionary steps wherever possible.

Frequently Asked Questions

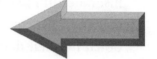

Q. If I go to the doctor several times in a year for different reasons, do I pay the deductible more than once?

A. No. Once your approved Medicare Part B expenses exceed $100 in the calendar year you have met the deductible requirement. Any expenses incurred through December 31 of the same year will be applied against the same $100.

Q. What is the difference between a deductible and co-insurance?

A. Deductibles are fixed dollar amounts that are paid by the patient in a specified Benefit Period. The amount is applied against the initial expenses incurred in that period.

Co-insurance is a means of sharing the cost of specific charges. It is paid by the patient against specific and individual services. Usually charged as a percentage of the cost incurred, it is in addition to any deductible.

Q. Can I get coverage for long-term care?

A. Private insurance companies sell long-term care insurance policies. Review them carefully before making any purchase. Terms, conditions, and prices vary widely among insurance companies. The premiums for these policies are now tax deductible.

Q. How do lifetime reserve days work?

A. Every person has 60 lifetime reserve days available to them to use for hospital stays. These are not renewable and can be used as needed at the patient's discretion. The daily co-insurance in 1998 is $382 per day. If a hospital stay exceeds 90 days, a patient can use lifetime reserve days for the additional hospital days. Once the 60 days are used up, there are no more available.

Q. What is an intermediate care facility?

A. These facilities provide care that is a step below a skilled nursing facility (SNF). They usually have medical and rehabilitation services available, but they do not provide the same level of daily care that is provided by SNFs.

Q. Does Medicare pay for intermediate care facilities?

A. No. Medicare will not pay the daily room and board charges. Costs for specific rehabilitative therapy received in an intermediate care facility may be paid by Medicare Part B if medical necessity is shown. The same is true of medical care rendered.

Q. If my doctor accepts assignment, what will I have to pay?

A. Your deductible and the 20 percent Part B co-insurance amount.

Q. **What happens if I am in the hospital for more than 90 days in one Benefit Period?**

A. Medicare's hospital coverage runs out on the 90th day. If you have lifetime reserve days available, you can use them. If you don't have any lifetime reserve days available, you are responsible for all hospital costs.

Q. **If I am out of the hospital for 60 days and go back in for treatment of the same illness, is this a new Benefit Period?**

A. Yes. Benefit Periods are counted by days between hospital or skilled nursing facility stays.

Q. **Are there deductibles for hospice care?**

A. No. There are no deductibles for hospice care for terminal illness. The patient pays only a small co-pay for prescription drugs. If the patient needs medical care for something not related to the terminal illness, the regular Medicare deductibles and co-insurance amounts apply.

Q. **If I don't have Medicare Part B, are my doctor's costs covered in the hospital?**

A. No. Doctor's services are a Medicare Part B expense.

Q. **What expenses will Medicare cover in a skilled nursing facility (SNF)?**

A. All the daily charges are covered for 100 days per Benefit Period. To be covered there must be medical necessity and the inpatient stay must start within 30 days of a three day hospitalization. For days 21 to 100, the patient must pay a $95.50 per day co-pay. After 100 days, there is no coverage.

CHAPTER **15**

Financial Self-Defense

Where to Begin? Medical expenses can mount very rapidly and without warning. Anyone who has ever reviewed a hospital bill line item by line item is amazed at the number of people who treated or came in contact with the patient, and at the charges for things you never noticed or heard of while being a patient yourself.

When you are in the midst of dealing with a serious medical crisis—either your own or that of someone you love—it is probably too late to try to deal with the cost issue. It is unlikely that any of us would withhold treatment while we wait for a cost estimate, which is all the more reason to be thoroughly familiar with your exposure before a crisis looms. You don't want to be burdened with this worry as well.

Three areas need to be addressed:

- How to pay for ongoing general medical care for maintaining good health and/or for the treatment of existing illnesses

- How to pay for serious acute illnesses, such as those requiring hospitalization or rehabilitation

- How to pay for needed long-term care

You may never need to deal with all three situations, but you should give some thought to each one. Before being able to make a proper judgment call about what kind of coverage you should have in addition to Medicare, you need to decide how much of your financial future you are willing to place at risk and how that would affect your spouse or other family members if the worst case were to happen. Answering the following questions will help provide a basis for decision making.

- How good is your current health?

- Do you smoke or engage in other activities that could have a long-term negative effect on your health?

- What is your current financial situation?

- What will be your future financial situation (in five years, ten years, 20 years) and how secure is it?

- What types and amounts of medical insurance coverage do you currently have?

- What premiums do you pay annually for each type of coverage?

- How much can you afford to spend on medical insurance annually?

- How much can you afford to pay for medical costs without jeopardizing your finances?

- If needed, are there other financial resources available within your family to help with medical bills?

- Is there anyone who could provide long-term care in the home for you?

- Do you have any idea what such care would cost?

- If you are relying on being taken care of by a child, what kind of effect would caring for you in this way have on his/her life or on his/her family's life?

- Are you being realistic about your choice of caretaker and have you discussed the possibility with the person you are thinking of?

- What effect would the costs of nursing home care have on your finances and the finances of other members of the family?

These are tough issues to think about. And these questions will probably lead you to others. This review isn't one that is easily undertaken and it is one that most people will happily put off. Maybe it isn't quite as bad as doing your taxes, but it is probably right up there on the list of things you'd rather avoid. The issues involved are emotional ones for all of us. Our health and our finances are very personal issues.

The Possibilities

Gaps and omissions in Medicare can cause you financial distress. Paying for long-term custodial care is among the costliest omissions, but the cost of managing a long-term illness can be equally burdensome.

There are no easy answers. There are no absolutely right answers because no one can foresee the future. Rather than just shouldering the risk or ignoring it, however, there are some things you can do.

▨ Unconventional Ideas

Protect your health as best you can. This step is entirely within your control. Do everything you can to stay healthy. If you stay reasonably healthy, your financial risk is drastically reduced because you won't have high medical bills. This might sound a bit odd as financial advice, but from a financial stand-point what is better than avoiding costs?

Caring for your health and protecting against health risks is within everyone's control. It is probably the only type of risk management that is.

Another unconventional way to reduce your out-of-pocket costs is to discuss fees with your doctor. No one likes to do it, but everyone else seems to be doing it—politicians, Medicare carriers, hospital administrators, insurance companies, and corporations. So the way has been paved for us, as patients, to open this kind of discussion with our doctors.

We all may be very reluctant to discuss costs, but medical treatment costs so much that our ability to pay for it may have to play a part in our decision about which treatment to have. Maybe it shouldn't, but the reality is that out-of-pocket costs can be sizable and need to be addressed before they become an insurmountable burden to the patient and his/her family.

Doctors are probably more familiar with the issue of medi-cal cost containment than just about anyone, so the topic probably won't be a shock to the doctor. Also, insurance compa-nies negotiate fees with doctors all the time, so why shouldn't you as a patient have the same opportunity?

There are three ways to "negotiate" fees:

1. Only use Medicare participating doctors. If your doctor is a participating doctor, your work is already done for you. Participating doctors must accept assignment for all claims. You don't have to negotiate, you just have to ask if the doctor is a participating physician.

In some states, such as Massachusetts, doctors are required to accept assignment as part of the licensing regulations. Other states are looking into adopting this practice as a consumer protection for patients. You can get a list of the participating physicians in your state by writing to the Medicare carrier in your area. (A complete listing of these is in Appendix A.)

2. Ask your doctor if s/he will accept assignment on some or all of your claims. When a physician or supplier agrees to assignment, he/she agrees to accept the Medicare approved amount. You will be responsible only for the co-insurance payment and deductibles. And your co-payment percentage will be calculated on the Medicare approved amount.

3. Discuss his/her fees with your doctor and see if you can limit your costs. This is probably the most difficult way to deal with the issue, but if you can be comfortable having this discussion you should.

Conventional Ideas

The other ways to fill in some of the gaps are:

- Buy a Medigap policy. This coverage will pay for deductibles, co-payments, outpatient prescriptions, and some other costs. You can choose among a number of policies with various amounts of coverage.

- Join a managed care program (e.g., HMO) that provides some of the missing coverage.

- Take advantage of an employer-sponsored health care program, if possible, if it provides better or additional coverage.

- Explore the available insurance options to pay for long-term care.

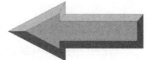

Frequently Asked Questions

Q. What does it mean when a physician accepts assignment?

A. The physician or supplier agrees not to charge you more than the Medicare approved amount for services and supplies covered by Part B. The physician is paid directly by Medicare, except for the deductible and co-insurance amounts for which you are responsible.

Q. How does the fee-for-service system work?

A. This is the traditional way to receive medical care. Under a fee-for-service system you can choose any physician, any hospital, any health care provider, or any facility approved by Medicare that agrees to accept you as a patient. A fee is charged each time you are treated and Medicare pays for its portion of the approved hospital, physician, or other health care expenses.

Q. Are there options for obtaining care under Medicare?

A. Yes. Medicare provides coverage under two different types of service plans:

1. Traditional fee-for-service (pay-as-you-go) plans and

2. Managed care plans, such as health maintenance organizations (HMOs), which have contracts with Medicare.

Both systems of medical care deliver comparable Medicare benefits. They differ in what medical services are covered, how and when payment is made, and how much you might have to pay out of your pocket.

Q. Do Medicare beneficiaries pay anything out of their own pockets when they use covered services?

A. Yes. With the traditional fee-for-service plan, both Part A and Part B have deductible and co-insurance amounts for which you are liable. You also must pay all permissible charges in excess of Medicare's approved amounts for Part B services, and all charges for services not covered by Medicare.

In a managed care plan, you usually make small co-payments when you obtain care.

Q. How do I find a Medicare participating physician or supplier?

A. All current Medicare participating physicians and suppliers are in the Medicare Participating Physician/Supplier Directory. This directory's listings are divided into geographic areas; the directory is available free of charge from your Medicare carrier (listed in Appendix A). If you don't want to wait to receive it, you can also call your carrier and ask for the names of some participating physicians and suppliers in your area. Most Social Security offices should also have a copy available for review.

Q. **If a physician is not a participating doctor, is there a limit to the amount s/he can charge a Medicare beneficiary for a covered service?**

A. Yes. Physicians who do not accept assignment of a Medicare claim are limited as to the amount they can charge Medicare beneficiaries for covered services. Charges by non-participating doctors for visits and consultations are capped at a percentage above Medicare's prevailing charge. This amount is shown on the EOMB.

Q. **Does Medicare pay for long-term care in a nursing home?**

A. No. Medicare only pays for extended care in a skilled nursing facility (SNF). And it only pays for 100 days of SNF coverage.

Nursing homes provide services that Medicare considers custodial. These are services that aid the patient in activities related to daily living that s/he cannot do without help.

Q. **Why does Medicare pay for skilled nursing facility care and not for nursing home care?**

A. Skilled nursing facilities provide daily medical care. All Medicare coverage hinges on proving that the treatment is medically necessary. When staff and equipment are used to provide skilled nursing care, rehabilitation therapies, or other health care services related to a particular medical condition that can be improved by this care, a case can be made for its medical necessity. If the care is mainly personal care or custodial services, such as help in walking, getting in and out of bed, eating, dressing, and bathing, it is not covered, even if the services are provided in a skilled nursing facility.

Q. Are any services covered for patients in nursing homes?

A. Yes. If you have a medical condition that is being treated by a doctor or you are receiving therapy, Medicare Part B may approve these expenses. It depends on what the care is and why you need it. But Medicare will not pay for the daily room and board charges of the nursing home.

Q. This seems confusing; how do the two preceding questions differ?

A. Medicare will only pay for the daily room and board charges in a skilled nursing facility when the care is medically necessary and is required every day. Payment for medical treatment in a nursing home is handled the same as if the patient were living on his/her own—payment is only made for the individual medical services.

Q. Does any federal program pay for nursing home care?

A. Yes. Medicaid may pay for nursing home care. The program varies by state; it is a program for people with little income and few assets. Many people who have assets before requiring long-term care end up covered by Medicaid because of the high cost of long-term care.

Q. Will long-term care insurance solve the problem?

A. Long-term care policies are sold by private insurance companies and vary widely in their coverage. They provide one way to protect against some of the costs of nursing home care, but the terms of the policy need to be examined carefully before choosing one.

Q. What if a physician or supplier will not accept assignment of a Medicare claim?

A. S/he may charge more than the Medicare approved amount and can collect payment directly from you. Medicare will reimburse you based on its approved amount, not the amount charged. You are liable for all permissible (there are certain limitations) charges in excess of Medicare's approved amount. You are also free to choose another medical provider before obtaining treatment.

Q. If I am in a skilled nursing facility, what happens after 100 days of Medicare coverage?

A. You pay all the costs.

Q. If Medicaid will cover the cost of nursing home care, why should I worry?

A. This depends on whether you have a spouse or someone who will still need to rely on your finances to live decently. Medicaid requires you to spend almost all of your money first.

CHAPTER **16**

Dealing With
Long-Term Care

**Defining
the
Question**

When we speak of long-term care, we cover a lot of ground. Generally we immediately think of nursing home care. But what is long-term care, really? We could reasonably argue that all of the following situations also qualify as types of long-term care:

- a several-month stay in a hospital or intermediate care facility

- a year of assisted recuperation at home

- months of rehabilitation in a skilled care facility

- staying in an assisted living facility

- living with a family member who takes care of most daily life chores

- hospice care for the terminally ill

My point is that long-term care is a complicated issue. The one thing that is clear in the situation is that Medicare won't be much help with paying for any of these situations, except perhaps, the hospice care.

Long-term care, whether it is custodial or medically necessary or somewhere in the grey area between the two, is expensive. Very expensive. And some of us are going to require it in one form or another. So how do we cut our risk?

First Things First

Think about what would happen if you suddenly required long-term care tomorrow. Can your family cope with it financially or practically? Can they cope with some of it? Can you pay for it? For how long? If your resources all go to your care, what happens to your spouse? What will Medicare cover?

These aren't happy questions and they don't have easy answers. Solid financial resources and/or insurance will help alleviate the worry and protect your family.

For most people the choices are:

■ At-home care provided by a family member—not ideal for a lot of reasons, but most of us would probably like to think we could provide it for our family members.

■ Inpatient rehabilitative care—expensive, and continual progress has to be shown to keep you in the facility.

■ Living on your own with live-in assistance—expensive, and good help is tough to find.

■ Using the services of an adult day care center—expensive.

■ Nursing home care—expensive.

So the issue boils down to protecting against the costs of hiring caregivers, or paying for a nursing home or intermediate care facility. Medicare may pay for some of the services needed. Insurance companies sell policies for long-term care. And Medicaid may be available after all other options are exhausted. (Medicare and Medicaid were more fully discussed in previous chapters, so we'll concentrate on long-term care insurance here.)

The Odds

In evaluating your risk of incurring long-term care costs, consider some information from the Census Bureau. For 1990–91, the percentage of people needing assistance with activities of daily living (bathing, cooking, personal care, etc.) ranged from nine percent of those age 65 to 69, to 50 percent of those age 85 or older. And people over 85 are the fastest-growing population segment in the country. This population increased 18.5 percent between 1990 and 1995 alone.

For those now aged 65 or older, estimates are that one in three people will spend three or more months in a nursing home; one in four will spend more than a year. Of course, the flip side of these figures is that two out of three people will spend less than three months in a nursing home.

As to the future and any individual's situation, who knows? There is absolutely no way to predict future health needs.

In the final analysis, buying insurance is a financial decision. If you can't afford long-term care coverage, don't let someone talk you into it. But if you have assets to protect and can afford it, it's wise to consider insurance. In making your decision, bear in mind that once you have an illness requiring long-term care, it will be too late to buy insurance to cover the costs.

Long-Term Care Insurance

If you do choose to explore private insurance protection, you have a difficult process ahead of you. There seem to be as many policy types and coverage choices as there are companies selling them. But the good news is that long-term care insurance is now partially deductible on your federal taxes.

Before exploring this area, think about what types of long-term care coverage you want to buy and how much you are willing or able to spend. As with all insurance purchases, it is important to be clear about what you are shopping for and to stick with that decision during the sales pitch.

The language of long-term care policies may be even more confusing than that of Medicare. Let's look at some of the different issues involved because they all affect the cost of the policy.

Waiver of premium — If you become ill and start receiving long-term care, this option allows you to stop paying any additional premiums.

Non-forfeiture benefits — This option returns some of your investment in the policy should you choose to drop the policy without ever using any of the benefits. The terms of these options vary by company and policy.

Death benefits — This option can result in a payment to your estate in the event of your death.

Inflation protection — Medical costs are constantly rising. If the policy does not account for increases over time, the benefit you pay for may be worth very little by the time you need it.

Long-term Care Worksheet

Item	Policy 1	Policy 2	Policy 3
Insurance company			
A. M. Best rating			
Annual/monthly cost			
Illness exclusions			
Pre-existing condition exclusions			
Deductibles			
Co-insurance			
Benefit type (daily payment, percentage payment)			
Benefit amount for nursing home care			
Benefit amount for home care			
Annual or lifetime maximum dollar benefit			
Annual or lifetime maximum number of months of coverage			
Waiting (or elimination) period before benefits begin			
Inflation protection to cover increases in costs			
Non-forfeiture benefit			
Death benefit			
Waiver of premiums once you receive care			
Is prior hospitalization required?			
Types of care covered			

Elimination periods — This is the waiting period before any benefits are paid.

Types of coverage — Coverage can range from skilled to intermediate to custodial care. It may pay only for care provided by licensed home health care agencies. It may be inpatient only or provide for home care as well. Clearly understanding the definition of the types of care covered by a policy is vital.

Type of benefit payment — Benefits can be paid as a daily fixed amount or a percentage of costs. Check on how this changes over time to protect against medical cost increases.

If you are unsure of any terminology when reviewing actual policies, insist that the terms be made clear for you before purchasing any insurance. Unlike Medigap or managed care, there are no government standards about coverage, so there is no easy way to compare policies. The worksheet at left will help you sort through the options and the questions to ask.

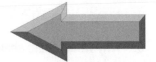

Frequently Asked Questions

Q. What kind of long-term care does Medicare pay for?

A. Medicare only pays for care in a skilled nursing facility and for a maximum of 100 days per Benefit Period.

Q. Doesn't Medicare pay for home health care services?

A. Yes, but only for limited medical services. Medicare does not cover assistance with housekeeping and other activities of daily living.

Q. Why get insurance if Medicaid will cover the costs?

A. Medicaid is for the poor; to qualify you have to have very few assets and little or no income. If you have assets and/or income you will have to spend almost all of it on your care before Medicaid will cover anything. Even with recent changes in the law, a spouse would be left in difficult circumstances under the Medicaid financial requirements.

Q. What are some of the options for long-term care?

A. Options include adult day care, live-in assistance, nursing home care, inpatient care in an intermediate or skilled nursing facility, daily homemaker or home health aide services, and home health care provided by licensed health care agencies.

Q. What kind of inflation protection should an insurance policy have?

A. The policy needs to contain a provision that allows you either to purchase additional coverage at specified times and additional premiums, or have a built-in inflation protector that increases your benefits automatically over time.

Q. Why would I care about a waiver of premiums?

A. If you are in a position to need long-term care, the chances are that your income and ability to pay the premiums would suffer. The waiver protects against a policy cancellation caused by such a circumstance.

Q. Where can I get additional information about long-term care policies?

A. Start by contacting your state's Department of Insurance and ask for general information. The state agencies on aging can refer you to information also, and they have insurance counseling services. Check Appendix D for contact addresses and phone numbers.

Q. How do I check on an insurance company that is trying to sell me a policy?

A. Contact your state's Insurance Department for information on companies licensed to do business in your state. Also check the A. M. Best insurance reference in your local library, which will give you financial information and assigns ratings to insurance companies.

CHAPTER 17

Evaluating Your Options

Making the Right Choice

Individual circumstances vary so widely that there is no perfect answer to the question of what to do about Medicare's gaps. I hope the information in this book has helped to clarify your questions and has provided the information you need to make decisions with which you are comfortable.

Financial surprises like uninsured medical costs are best avoided, if possible. By learning about Medicare and looking at your options, you will lessen the possibility of an unpleasant surprise.

In making your decision, consider the following steps to help find the right answer for you and your family.

1. Review your current financial situation.

    - How much can you afford to pay for insurance policies, based on your income?

    - How much can you afford to spend on out-of-pocket medical expenses before your lifestyle is compromised?

    - How dependable is your income?

2. Find out what types of policies are available in your area.

    - Are Medicare managed care plans available?

218

- What types of Medigap policies are available?

- What types of long-term care policies are available?

3. Decide which assets and income need protecting and for whom.

  - Do you have dependents who rely on your income?

  - What assets do you and your spouse need to maintain your lifestyle?

  - How will your spouse manage if some medical catastrophe strikes?

4. Decide what your tolerance for risk is.

  - How much risk can you afford to assume?

  - How much risk of incurring medical costs are you comfortable with?

  - What are the consequences, financially and personally, if the worst situation happens?

5. Review your options for affordability and for how they fit in with your lifestyle.

  - How much flexibility in choosing doctors do you want?

  - What is the current state of your health and how confident are you about maintaining a good level of health in the future?

  - Do you have pre-existing conditions that may make purchasing insurance difficult later?

  - Does your travel schedule or having a second residence limit your coverage choices?

6. Think about your comfort level with the company proposing to sell you the policy.

   ■ Are you satisfied that you have had all your questions fully answered?

   ■ Have you checked the company's A. M. Best rating?

   ■ Are you satisfied with the type and scope of the coverage?

   ■ Are you clear about any exclusions contained in the policy?

   ■ Have you received quotes from a few different companies to compare prices?

7. Explore all the issues.

   ■ If you have assets to protect, have you consulted with an attorney specializing in trusts or in elder care law?

   ■ Do you know what the Medicaid requirements are in your state, so that you fully understand what would happen financially to you or your spouse in a worst case scenario?

These questions will lead to others as you go through the review process. Take your time and don't let yourself be pushed into any one insurance policy or solution. Trying to deal with your future financial health requires a lot of thought, and the information won't be gathered overnight. If you set a time frame for making a decision and stick to it, you will be able to accomplish your goal without undue haste.

Appendix

- Sections A through I list the names, addresses and phone numbers for agencies that can offer information and counseling on Medicare and other related issues.

- Section K defines commonly used insurance terms.

Phone numbers for government agencies sometimes seem to have a life of their own and they change fairly frequently. Toll-free numbers particularly tend to appear and disappear based on budgets, so don't be surprised if a toll-free number has been disconnected. Don't give up, even if you run into the occasional person who will be unfriendly or unhelpful. Most people in these agencies are willing to be helpful, but you need to be as clear as possible about the information you require so that they can refer you to the right person.

SECTION A

Medicare Carriers and Intermediaries

Alabama

Medicare
Blue Cross & Blue Shield
 of Alabama
450 Riverchase Parkway East
Birmingham, AL 35298
205-988-2244
800-292-8855

Alaska

Medicare Part B Claims
Blue Cross & Blue Shield
 of North Dakota
P.O. Box 6703
Fargo, ND 58108-6703
800-444-4606

Arizona

Medicare Part B
Blue Cross & Blue Shield of
 North Dakota
P.O. Box 6704
Fargo, ND 58108-6704
800-444-4606

Arkansas

Medicare
Arkansas Blue Cross &
 Blue Shield
601 Gaines Street
Little Rock, AR 72203
501-378-2000
800-482-5525 (Arkansas only)

California (North)

Medicare Service
NHIC – National Heritage
 Insurance Company
Chico, CA 95976
916-743-1583
800-952-8627 (CA only)
530-634-7538 (TTY)

California (South)

Medicare Part A
Blue Cross of California
Box 9140
Camarillo, CA 93031
818-593-2006

222

Medicare Part B
Transamerica Life Company
P.O. Box 54905
Los Angeles, CA 90054-0905
213-748-2311
800-675-2266 (Southern
   California only)

Colorado
Medicare
Blue Cross & Blue Shield
   of North Dakota
4305 13th Avenue SW
Fargo, ND 58103
701-282-1100
800-444-4606

Connecticut
Medicare
P.O. Box 9000
538 Preston Avenue
Meriden, CT 06450
203-639-3000
203-237-8592
800-982-6819 (Connecticut only)

Delaware
Claims
Xact Medicare Services Part B
P.O. Box 890065
Camp Hill, PA 17089-0065
General Information
P.O. Box 890413
Camp Hill, PA 17089-0413
717-763-3151
800-851-3535 (Delaware only)
800-242-8471 (TDD)

District of Columbia
Xact Medicare Claims Services
P.O. Box 890065
Camp Hill, PA 17089-0065
General Information
P.O. Box 890413
Camp Hill, PA 17089-0413
717-763-3151
800-233-1124 (District of
   Columbia)
800-242-8471 (TDD)

Florida
Medicare
Blue Cross & Blue Shield
   of Florida, Inc.
P.O. Box 2078
Jacksonville, FL 32231
904-791-6111
800-333-7586 (Florida only)

Georgia
Medicare Part B
Cahaba Government
   Benefits Administrators
P.O. Box 3018
Savannah, GA 31402-3018
912-920-2412
800-727-0827

Hawaii
Medicare Part B
Blue Cross & Blue Shield
   of North Dakota
P.O. Box 6701
Fargo, ND 58108-6701
800-444-4606

Idaho

Medicare
CIGNA
Two Vantage Way
Nashville, TN 37228
615-244-5600
800-627-2782 (Idaho only)

Illinois

Medicare Part A Claims
Health Care Service Corp.
300 Randolph Street
Chicago, IL 60690
Medicare Part B Claims
Health Care Service Corp.
P.O. Box 5533
Marion, IL 62959
312-938-8000
800-642-6930 (outside 312)
800-535-6152 (TDD)

Indiana

Medicare
Associated Insurance Co.
8115 Knue Road
Indianapolis, IN 46250
317-841-4400
800-622-4792

Iowa

Medicare
Wellmark, Inc.
636 East Grand Avenue,
 Station 28
Des Moines, IA 50309
515-245-4618
800-532-1285

Kansas

Medicare Parts A & B
Blue Cross and Blue Shield
 of Kansas
P.O. Box 239
1133 SW Topeka Boulevard
Topeka, KS 66629-0001
913-291-7000
800-432-3531 (Kansas only)
800-432-0216

Kentucky

Medicare
Adminastar Federal
d/b/a Blue Cross & Blue
 Shield of Kentucky
9901 Linn Station Road
Louisville, KY 40223
502-425-6759
502-329-8559
800-999-7608

Louisiana

Medicare
Arkansas Blue Cross
 & Blue Shield
P.O. Box 98501
Baton Rouge, LA 70884
504-927-3490
800-462-9666 (Louisiana only)
504-231-2292 (TDD)

Maine

Medicare
National Heritage Insurance Co.
NHIC-NE
P.O. Box 1000

Hingham, MA 02044
800-492-0919
800-668-1339 (TDD)

Maryland
Medicare
Trailblazers Health Enterprises
11350 McCormick Road
Executive Plaza 3
Hunt Valley, MD 21031
Claims
P.O. Box 5798
Timonium, MD 21094-5798
800-444-4606
800-516-6684 (TDD)

Massachusetts
Medicare
National Heritage Insurance
 Company
P.O. Box 1000
Hingham, MA 02044
800-882-1228
800-668-1339 (TDD)

Michigan
Medicare Part A
Health Care Service Corp.
300 Randolph Street
Chicago, IL 60690
Medicare Part B
Health Care Service Corp.
P.O. Box 5533
Marion, IL 62959
312-938-8000
800-642-6930
800-535-6152 (TDD)

Minnesota
*Counties of Anoka, Dakota,
Fillmore, Goodhue, Hennepin,
Houston, Olmstead, Ramsey,
Wabasha, Washington, and
Winona:*
Minnesota Medicare
The Travelers Insurance Co.
8120 Penn Avenue
South Bloomington, MN
 55431-1394
612-885-2800
800-352-2762 (Minnesota
 only)

All other counties:
Medicare
Blue Cross & Blue Shield
 of Minnesota
P.O. Box 64560
St. Paul, MN 55164-0560
Claims
P.O. Box 64338
St. Paul, MN 55164-0338
612-456-8000
800-382-2000 x5503
888-878-0136 (TDD)

Mississippi
Medicare
United Health Care
P.O. Box 22545
Jackson, MS 39225-2545
601-956-0372
800-682-5417 (Mississippi
 only)
601-977-5820 (TDD)

Missouri

Counties of Andrew, Atchison, Bates, Benton, Buchanan, Caldwell, Carroll, Cass, Clay, Clinton, Daviess, DeKalb, Gentry, Grundy, Harrison, Henry, Holt, Jackson, Johnson, Lafayette, Livingston, Mercer, Nodaway, Pettis, Platte, Ray, St. Clair, Saline, Vernon, and Worth:

Medicare Part B
Blue Cross & Blue Shield
   of Kansas
1133 SW Topeka Boulevard
Topeka, KS 66629
785-291-4003
800-892-5900
800-430-8757 (TDD)

All other counties:

Medicare
General American Life
   Insurance Company
P.O. Box 505
St. Louis, MO 63166
314-843-8880
800-392-3070
314-525-6672 (TDD)
800-645-6672 (TDD)

Montana

Medicare
Blue Cross & Blue Shield
   of Montana
P.O. Box 4310
340 Last Chance Gulch
Helena, MT 59604
406-444-8350
800-332-6146 (Montana only)

Nebraska

Medicare
Blue Cross & Blue Shield
   of Kansas
1133 SW Topeka Boulevard
Topeka, KS 66629-0001
785-291-4155
800-633-1113 (Nebraska only)

Nevada

Medicare
Aetna Life & Casualty
   Company
4000 South Eastern Avenue,
   Suite 150
Las Vegas, NV 89119
702-659-8200
800-410-3015 (Nevada only)

New Hampshire

Medicare
National Heritage Insurance
   Company
P.O. Box 1000
Hingham, MA 02044
800-447-1142
800-668-1339 (TDD)

New Jersey

Xact Medicare Services
P.O. Box 890065
Camp Hill, PA 17089-0065
800-462-9306
800-992-0165 (TDD)

New Mexico
Medicare Part B
Blue Cross & Blue Shield
  of Arkansas
Regency Center Office Park
701 NW 63rd Street
Oklahoma City, OK 73116-
  7693
405-848-7711
800-522-9079 (Oklahoma
  only)
800-822-9472 (TDD)

New York
*Counties of Bronx, Columbia,
Delaware, Duchess, Greene,
Kings, Nassau, New York,
Orange, Putnam, Richmond,
Rockland, Suffolk, Sullivan,
Ulster, and Westchester:*
Medicare
Empire Blue Cross &
  Blue Shield
622 Third Avenue
New York, NY 10017
212-476-1000
800-442-8430 (New York
  only)
800-873-1322 (TDD)

All other counties:
Medicare
Blue Cross & Blue Shield
  of Western New York
P.O. Box 80
1901 Main Street
Buffalo, NY 14240-0080

716-887-6900
800-888-0757
716-884-2370 (TDD)

North Carolina
Medicare
CIGNA Medicare
7736 McCloud Road,
  Suite 240
Greensboro, NC 27409
910-665-0341
800-672-3071 (North
  Carolina only)

North Dakota
Medicare
Blue Cross & Blue Shield
  of North Dakota
P.O. Box 6706
Fargo, ND 58108-6706
701-277-2263
800-247-2267
800-659-3656 (TDD)

Ohio
Medicare Part B
Nationwide Mutual
  Insurance Company
One Nationwide Plaza
P.O. Box 57
Columbus, OH 43216
614-249-7157
800-282-0530 (Ohio only)
800-542-5250 (TDD)

Oklahoma

Medicare
Blue Cross & Blue Shield
of Arkansas
701 NW 63rd Street, 3rd
Floor
Oklahoma City, OK 73116-
7693
405-848-6257

Oregon

Medicare Part B Claims
Blue Cross & Blue Shield
of North Dakota
Box 6702
Fargo, ND 58108-6702
800-444-4606

Pennsylvania

Xact Medicare Services
P.O. Box 890065
Camp Hill, PA 17089-0065
800-382-1274
800-242-8471 (TDD)

Rhode Island

Medicare
Blue Cross & Blue Shield
of Rhode Island
444 Westminster Street
Providence, RI 02903-3279
401-861-2273
800-662-5170
401-459-1756 (TDD)
888-239-3356 (TDD)

South Carolina

Medicare
Blue Cross & Blue Shield
of South Carolina
d/b/a Palmetto Government
Benefits Administrators
300 Arbor Lake Drive,
Suite 800
Columbia, SC 29223
803-788-3882
800-868-2522
800-223-1296 (TDD)

South Dakota

Medicare
Blue Cross & Blue Shield
of North Dakota
P.O. Box 6707
Fargo, ND 58108-6707
701-277-2273
800-437-4762

Tennessee

Medicare
CIGNA Medicare
P.O. Box 1465
Nashville, TN 37202
615-244-5600
800-342-8900 (Tennessee
only)

Texas

Medicare

Blue Cross & Blue Shield
of Texas
901 South Central Expressway
Richardson, TX 75080
or

Medicare Part B Claims

Blue Cross & Blue Shield
of Texas
P.O. Box 660031
Dallas, TX 75266-0031
214-766-6900
800-442-2620
800-252-8012 (TDD)

Utah

Medicare
Blue Cross & Blue Shield
of Utah
P.O. Box 30270
Salt Lake City, UT 84130
801-487-6441
800-662-6515 (Utah only)

Vermont

Medicare
National Heritage Insurance
Company
P.O. Box 1000
Hingham, MA 02044
800-447-1142
800-668-1339 (TDD)

Virginia

Medicare
United Health Care
P.O. Box 26463
Richmond, VA 23261
300 Arboretum Place
Richmond, VA 23236
804-300-4786
804-330-6100
800-552-3423 (Virginia only)

Washington

Medicare Part B
Blue Cross & Blue Shield
of North Dakota
P.O. Box 6700
Fargo, ND 58108-6700
800-444-4606
800-377-4950 (TDD)

West Virginia

Medicare Operations
Department
Nationwide Mutual
Insurance Company
P.O. Box 57
Columbus, OH 43216
800-848-0106 (West
Virginia only)
800-542-5250 (TDD)

Wisconsin

Medicare
Wisconsin Physicians'
  Services Insurance Corp.
P.O. Box 1787
Madison, WI 53701
608-221-4711
800-944-0051 (Wisconsin
  only)
800-828-2837 (TDD)

Wyoming

Medicare
Blue Cross & Blue Shield
  of North Dakota
711 2nd Avenue
Fargo, ND 58102
800-437-4762

Puerto Rico

Medicare
Triple-S, Inc.
P.O. Box 71391
San Juan, PR 00936
or
Medicare
Triple-S, Inc.
1441 F. D. Roosevelt Avenue
Puerto Neuvo, PR 00921
787-749-4080

Virgin Islands

Medicare
Triple-S, Inc.
P. O. Box 363628
San Juan, PR 00936-3628
787-749-4949, ext. 4438

SECTION B

Nursing Home Licensing Agencies

Alabama

Nursing Home Licensure
  Office
Division of Licensure
  and Certification
Alabama Department
  of Public Health
201 Monroe Street
RSA Tower, Suite 600
Montgomery, AL 36104
Mail:
P.O. Box 303017
Montgomery, AL 36130-3017
334-206-5100

Alaska

Department of Health
  and Social Services
Health Facilities Licensing
  and Certification
4730 Business Park Boule-
  vard, Suite 18
Anchorage, AK 99503
907-561-8081

Arizona

Department of Health
  Services
Office of Health Care
  Licensure
1647 East Morton
  Avenue, Suite 100
Phoenix, AZ 85020
602-255-1177

Arkansas

Department of Human
  Services
Certification and
  Licensure Section
Office of Long Term
  Care
P.O. Box 8059, Slot 404
Little Rock, AR 72203-
  8059
501-682-8430

California

Nursing Home Licensure
Office
Licensure and Certification
Division
Facilities Licensing Section
P.O. Box 942732
1800 3rd Street, Suite 210
Sacramento, CA 94234-7320
916-445-2070

Colorado

Colorado Department
of Public Health and
Environment
Environment Health
Facilities Division
4300 Cherry Creek Drive
South
Denver, CO 80246
303-692-2800

Connecticut

Nursing Home Licensure
Office
Department of Public
Health
Division of Health System
Regulation
410 Capitol Avenue,
MS #12 HFL
P.O. Box 340308
Hartford, CT 06134
860-509-7444

Delaware

Office of Health Facilities
Licensing and Certification
Nursing Home Division
Division of Public Health
3 Mill Road, Suite 308
Wilmington, DE 19806
302-577-6666

District of Columbia

Office of Licensing and
Certification
Department of Consumer
and Regulatory Affairs
Service Facility Regulation
Administration
614 H Street NW, Suite 1003
Washington, DC 20001
202-727-7190

Florida

Nursing Home Licensure
Office
Licensure and Certification
Branch
Long Term Care Division
Agency of Health Care
Administration
2727 Mahan Drive, Bldg. 1
Tallahassee, FL 32308
850-488-5861

Georgia

Long Term Care Section
Office of Regulatory Services
2 Peachtree Street NW,
   Room 31-447
Atlanta, GA 30303-3167
404-657-5850

Hawaii

Hospital and Medical
   Facility Branch
1270 Queen Emma Street,
   Suite 1100
Honolulu, HI 96813
808-586-4090

Idaho

Bureau of Facilities
   Standards
Idaho Department of
   Health and Welfare
P.O. Box 83720
Boise, ID 83720-0036
208-334-6626

Illinois

Illinois Department of
   Public Health
Division of Long Term
   Care Quality Assurance
525 West Jefferson Street,
   5th Floor
Springfield, IL 62761
217-782-5180
800-547-0466 (TTY)

Indiana

Indiana State Department
   of Health
Division of Long Term Care
2 North Meridian Street,
   Section B
Indianapolis, IN 46204
317-233-7442

Iowa

Department of Inspections
   and Appeals
Division of Health Facilities
Lucas State Office Building,
   3rd Floor
Des Moines, IA 50319-0083
515-281-4115
515-242-6515 (TDD)

Kansas

Department of Health
   and Environment
Bureau of Adult and Child
   Care
900 SW Jackson, Suite 1001
Topeka, KS 66612-1290
785-296-1240
800-842-0078

Kentucky

Division for Licensing
   and Regulation
Office of the Inspector
   General
275 East Main Street, 4E-A
Frankfort, KY 40621
502-564-2800

Louisiana

Department of Health
and Hospitals
Health Standards Section
P.O. Box 3767
Baton Rouge, LA 70821-3767
504-342-0148

Maine

Department of Human Services
Division of Licensure
and Certification
35 Anthony Avenue
State House Station 11
Augusta, ME 04333
207-624-5443

Maryland

Licensing and Certification
Administration
Department of Health
and Mental Hygiene
4201 Patterson Avenue, 4th Floor
Baltimore, MD 21215
410-764-2770
800-492-6005

Massachusetts

Long Term Care Facilities
Program
Department of Public Health
10 West Street, 5th Floor
Boston, MA 02111
617-753-8000
800-462-5531

Michigan

Department of Consumer
Industry Services
Bureau of Health Systems
525 West Ottawa
P.O. Box 30664
Lansing, MI 48909
517-334-8408

Minnesota

Department of Health
Health Resources Division
393 North Dunlop Street
P.O. Box 64900
St. Paul, MN 55164-0900
612-643-2100

Mississippi

Mississippi Department
of Health
Division of Licensure
and Certification
P.O. Box 1700
Jackson, MS 39215-1700
601-354-7300

Missouri

Department of Social
Services
Division of Aging
615 Howerton Court
Jefferson City, MO 65109
573-751-3082
800-735-2966 (TDD)

Montana

Department of Public
    Health and Human
    Services
Quality Assurance Division
Health Facilities Division
Licensure Bureau
Cogswell Building
1400 Broadway
P.O. Box 202951
Helena, MT 59620-2951
406-444-2037
406-444-2676 (Licensure)
406-444-2099 (Certification)

Nebraska

Facility Credentialing
Department of Health
    and Human Services
301 Centennial Mall, South
Lincoln, NE 68509-5007
402-471-2949
402-471-6421 (TDD)

Nevada

Human Resources
    Department
Health Administration
Bureau of Licensure and
    Certification
1550 East College Parkway,
    #158
Carson City, NV 89706
702-687-4475

New Hampshire

Department of Health
    and Human Serivces
Office of Program Support
Bureau of Health Facilities
    Administration
6 Hazen Drive
Concord, NH 03301-6527
603-271-4592
800-852-3345

New Jersey

NJ State Department of
    Health and Senior Services
Licensing CN367
120 S. Stockton Street
Trenton, NJ 08611
Mail:
P.O. Box 367
Trenton, NJ 08625-0367
609-633-9042
800-792-9770 (ask for
    licensing)

New Mexico

Health Facility Licensing
    and Certification Bureau
525 Camino de los Marquez,
    Suite 2
Santa Fe, NM 87501
505-827-4200

New York

Bureau of Long Term Care
  Services
New York State Department
  of Health
99 Washington Avenue,
  Suite 1126
Albany, NY 12210-2811
518-473-1564

North Carolina

Nursing Home Licensure
  Office
Licensure and Certification
  Section
Health Care Facilities Branch
701 Barbour Drive
Raleigh, NC 27603
919-733-7461
800-662-7030

North Dakota

Department of Health
Health Facilities Division
600 East Boulevard Avenue
Bismarck, ND 58505-0200
701-328-2352

Ohio

Division of Quality
  Assurance
Licensure Program
246 North High Street,
  3rd Floor
Columbus, OH 43266-0588
614-466-7713

Oklahoma

Special Health Services
Licensure and Certification
  Division
1000 NE 10th Street
Oklahoma City, OK 73117-
  1299
405-271-6868
800-747-8419

Oregon

Senior and Disabled Services
  Division
Long Term Care Licensing
Licensing and Certification
500 Summer Street NE
Salem, OR 97310
503-945-5833
800-422-6012 (Oregon only)

Pennsylvania

Pennsylvania Department
  of Health
Division of Nursing
Room 526, Health and
  Welfare Building
Harrisburg, PA 17120
Mail:
Nursing Home Licensure
  Office
Division of Nursing Care
  Facilities
P.O. Box 90
Harrisburg, PA 17108
717-787-1816

Rhode Island
Department of Health
Division of Facilities
    Regulation
3 Capitol Hill
Providence, RI 02908-5097
401-277-2566
401-277-2506 (TDD)

South Carolina
South Carolina Department
    of Health and Environ-
    mental Control
Bureau of Health Regulation
1777 St. Julian Place,
    Heritage Bldg.
Columbia, SC 29204
Mail:
South Carolina Department
    of Health and Environ-
    mental Control
Bureau of Health Regulation
2600 Bull Street
Columbia, SC 29201
803-737-7200

South Dakota
Department of Health
Licensure and Certification
615 East 4th
Pierre, SD 57501-1700
605-773-3356

Tennessee
Department of Health
Division of Health Care
    Facilities
Cordell Hull Building
425 Fifth Avenue North,
    1st Floor
Nashville, TN 37247-0508
615-741-7221

Texas
Department of Health
Licensing and Certification
    Bureau
1100 West 49th Street
Austin, TX 78756-3199
512-834-6650

Utah
Department of Health
Health Care Resources
Health Facilities Licensure
    Bureau
288 North 1460 West
Salt Lake City, UT 84116
Mail:
Department of Health
Health Care Resources
Health Facilities Licensure
    Bureau
Box 142853
Salt Lake City, UT 84114-
    2853
801-538-6152

Vermont
Aging and Disabilities
  Department
Licensing and Protection
  Division
103 S. Main Street
Ladd Hall
Waterbury, VT 05671-2306
802-241-2345
800-564-1612 (Vermont only)

Virginia
Center for Quality
  Health Care Services
  and Consumer Protection
Department of Health
3600 West Broad Street,
  Suite 216
Richmond, VA 23230-4920
804-367-2102
800-955-1819

Washington
Department of Health
1300 SE Quince Street
Olympia, WA 98504-0935
360-586-5846
800-525-0127

West Virginia
Health and Human
  Resources Department
Administration and
  Finance Bureau
Health Facilities and Licen-
  sure Certification Section
1900 Canal Blvd. East
Building 3, Room 550
Charleston, WV 25305
304-558-0050
800-442-2888 (West
  Virginia only)

Wisconsin
Health and Family
  Services Department
Division of Supported Living
Bureau of Quality Assurance
P.O. Box 309
Madison WI 53701
608-266-8481

Wyoming
Health Department
Division of Health
Office of Health Quality
First Bank Building,
  8th Floor
Cheyenne, WY 82002-0480
307-777-7123
307-777-5648 (TDD)

SECTION C

Peer Review Organizations

Alabama

Alabama Quality Assurance
  Foundation, Inc.
1 Perimeter Park South,
  Suite 200N
Birmingham, AL 35243-2354
205-970-1600
800-760-4550

Alaska

PRO-WEST
721 Sesame Street, Suite 1A
Anchorage, AK 99503
907-562-2252 (Anchorage
  only)
800-445-6941

Arizona

Health Services Advisory
  Group, Inc.
301 East Bethany Home
  Road, B-157
Phoenix, AZ 85012
602-264-6382
800-626-1577 (Arizona only)
800-359-9909

Arkansas

Arkansas Foundation for
  Medical Care, Inc.
2201 Broken Hill Drive
Fort Smith, AR 72908
Mail:
Arkansas Foundation for
  Medical Care, Inc.
P.O. Box 180001
Fort Smith, AR 72918-0001
501-649-8501
800-272-5528 (Arkansas only)

California

California Medical Review,
  Inc.
60 Spear Street, Suite 400
San Francisco, CA 94105
415-882-5800
800-841-1602 (California
  only)
800-881-5980 (TDD)

Colorado

Colorado Foundation
  for Medical Care
2851 South Parker Road,
  Suite 200
Aurora, CO 80014
or
Colorado Foundation
  for Medical Care
P.O. Box 17300
Denver, CO 80217-0300
303-695-3300
800-727-7086 (Colorado
  only)
303-695-3314 (TDD)

Connecticut

Connecticut Peer Review
  Organization, Inc.
100 Roscommon Drive,
  Suite 200
Middletown, CT 06457
860-632-2008
800-553-7590 (Connecticut
  only)

Delaware

West Virginia Medical
  Institute, Inc.
3001 Chesterfield Place
Charleston, WV 25304
304-346-9864
800-642-8686

District of Columbia

Delmarva Foundation
  for Medical Care, Inc.
9240 Centreville Road
Easton, MD 21601
410-822-0697
800-645-0011 (DC only)

Florida

Florida Medical Quality
  Assurance, Inc.
4350 West Cypress Street,
  Suite 900
Tampa, FL 33607
813-354-9111
800-844-0795

Georgia

Georgia Medical Care
  Foundation
57 Executive Park South, NE
Suite 200
Atlanta, GA 30329
404-982-0411
800-282-2614 (Georgia only)

Hawaii

Hawaii Medical Service
  Association
818 Keeaumoku Street
P.O. Box 860
Honolulu, HI 96808-0860
808-948-6111
800-776-4672
808-948-6222 (TDD)

Idaho

PRO-WEST
815 Park Blvd., Suite 250
Boise, ID 83712
208-343-4617
800-488-1118

Illinois

Illinois Foundation for
  Quality Health Care
6000 Westown Parkway,
  Suite 350
West Des Moines, IA 50266-
  7771
515-223-2900
800-647-8089

Indiana

Health Care Excel
2901 Ohio Boulevard
P.O. Box 3713
Terre Haute, IN 47803-3713
800-288-1499

Iowa

Iowa Foundation for Medi-
  cal Care
6000 Westown Parkway,
  Suite 350E
West Des Moines, IA 50266-
  7771
515-223-2900
800-752-7014

Kansas

The Kansas Foundation
  for Medical Care, Inc.
2947 SW Wanamaker Drive
Topeka, KS 66614
913-273-2552
800-432-0407

Kentucky

Health Care Excel
9502 Williamsburg Plaza,
  #102
Louisville, KY 40222
800-288-1499

Louisiana

Louisiana Health Care
  Review, Inc.
8591 United Plaza Boulevard,
  Suite 270
Baton Rouge, LA 70809
504-926-6353
800-433-4958 (Louisiana
  only)

Maine

Northeast Healthcare
  Quality Foundation
15 Old Rollinsford Road,
  Suite 302
Dover, NH 03820
603-749-1641
800-772-0151 (New England
  only)

Maryland

Delmarva Foundation
  for Medical Care, Inc.
9240 Centreville Road
Easton, MD 21601
410-822-0697
800-645-0011
800-492-5811 (Maryland
  only)

Massachusetts

Massachusetts Peer Review
  Organization, Inc.
235 Wyman Street
Waltham, MA 02154-1231
781-890-0011 (call collect
  from out of state)
800-252-5533 (Massachusetts
  only)

Michigan

Michigan Peer Review
  Organization
40600 Ann Arbor Road,
  Suite 200
Plymouth, MI 48170-4495
735-459-0900
800-365-5899
800-649-3777 (TDD)

Minnesota

Stratus Health
2901 Metro Drive, Suite 400
Bloomington, MN 55425
612-854-3306
800-444-3423 (Minnesota
  only)

Mississippi

Mississippi Foundation
  for Medical Care, Inc.
735 Riverside Drive
P.O. Box 4665
Jackson, MS 39296-4665
601-948-8894
800-844-0600

Missouri

Missouri Patient Care
  Review Foundation
505 Hobbs Road, Suite 100
Jefferson City, MO 65109
573-893-7900
800-347-1016

Montana

Mountain Pacific Quality
  Health Foundation
400 North Park, 2nd Floor
Helena, MT 59601
406-443-4020
800-497-8232

Nebraska

Iowa Foundation for
  Medical Care
The Sunderbruch Corpora-
  tion (NE)
1221 N Street, Suite 800
CTU Building
Lincoln, NE 68508
402-474-7471
800-247-3004 (Nebraska
  only)

Nevada

Health Insight
901 South Rancho Lane,
Suite 200
Las Vegas, NV 89106
702-385-9933 (call collect
from out of state)
800-748-6773

North Dakota

North Dakota Health Care
Review, Inc.
800 31st Avenue SW
Minot, ND 58701
701-852-4231
800-472-2902

New Hampshire

Northeast Healthcare Quality
Foundation
15 Old Rollinsford Road,
Suite 302
Dover, NH 03820
603-749-1641 (call collect
from out of state)
800-772-0151 (New England
only)

New Jersey

The Peer Review Organization
of New Jersey, Inc.
Central Division
Brier Hill Court, Building J
East Brunswick, NJ 08816
732-238-5570 (call collect
from out of state)
800-624-4557 (New Jersey only)

New Mexico

New Mexico Medical Review
Association
2340 Menaul NE, Suite 300
Albuquerque, NM 87107
Mail:
P.O. Box 3200
Albuquerque, NM 87190-
3200
505-998-9898
505-842-6236 (Albuquerque
only)
800-432-6824 (New Mexico
only)

New York

Island Peer Review
Organization, Inc.
1979 Marcus Avenue,
1st Floor
Lake Success, NY 11042
516-326-7767 (call collect
from out of state)
800-331-7767

North Carolina

Medical Review of North
Carolina
5625 Dillard Drive, Suite 203
Cary, NC 27511-9227
919-851-2955
800-722-0468 (North and
South Carolina only)

Ohio
Peer Review Systems, Inc.
757 Brooksedge Plaza Drive
Westerville, OH 43081-4913
614-895-9900
800-589-7337 (Ohio only)
800-837-0664

Oklahoma
Foundation for Medical
  Quality
5801 Broadway Extension
The Paragon Building,
  Suite 400
Oklahoma City, OK 73118-
  9984
405-840-2891
800-522-3414 (Oklahoma
  only)

Oregon
Oregon Medical Professional
  Review Organization
2020 SW 4th Avenue,
  Suite 520
Portland, OR 97201-4960
503-279-0100
800-344-4354

Pennsylvania
Keystone Peer Review
  Organization, Inc.
777 East Park Drive
P.O. Box 8310
Harrisburg, PA 17105-8310
717-564-8288
800-322-1914

Rhode Island
Rhode Island Quality
  Partners
100 Roscommon Drive, #200
Middletown, CT 06457
860-632-2008
800-662-5028

South Carolina
Carolina Medical Review
250 Berry Hill Road,
  Suite 101
Columbia, SC 29210
803-731-8225
800-922-3089 (South
  Carolina only)

South Dakota
South Dakota Foundation
  for Medical Care
1323 South Minnesota
  Avenue
Sioux Falls, SD 57105
605-336-3505
800-658-2285

Tennessee
Mid-South Foundation
  for Medical Care
6401 Poplar Avenue,
  Suite 400
Memphis, TN 38119
901-682-0381
800-489-4633

Texas

Texas Medical Foundation
Barton Oaks Plaza 2,
  Suite 200
901 Mopac Expressway
  South
Austin, TX 78746-5799
512-329-6610
800-725-8315 (Texas only)
800-725-8339 (TDD)

Utah

Health Insight
675 East 2100 South,
  Suite 270
Salt Lake City, UT 84106-
  1864
801-487-2290
800-274-2290

Vermont

New Hampshire Foundation
  for Medical Care
15 Old Rollinsford Road,
  Suite 302
Dover, NH 03820
603-749-1641
800-772-0151 (New England
  only)

Virginia

Medical Society of Virginia
  Review Organization
1606 Santa Rosa Road,
  Suite 200
P.O. Box K70
Richmond, VA 23288-0070
804-289-5397 (Richmond
  only)
800-545-3814 (Washington
  D.C., Maryland, and
  Virginia only)

Washington

PRO-WEST
10700 Meridian Avenue,
  North
Suite 100
Seattle, WA 98133-9075
206-364-9700
206-368-8272 (Seattle only)
800-445-6941

West Virginia

West Virginia Medical
  Institute, Inc.
3001 Chesterfield Place
Charleston, WV 25304
304-346-9864 (Charleston
  only)
800-642-8686

Wisconsin

Metastar/WIPRO
2909 Landmark Place
Madison, WI 53713
608-274-1940
800-362-2320 (Wisconsin
  only)
608-274-8350 (TDD)

Wyoming

Mountain Pacific Quality
  Health Foundation
400 North Park, 2nd Floor
Helena, MT 59601
406-443-4020
800-497-8232

Puerto Rico

Puerto Rico Foundation
  for Medical Care
Mercantile Plaza, Suite 605
Hato Rey, PR 00918
787-753-6705 (call collect
  from outside Puerto Rico)
800-981-5262 (Puerto Rico
  only)

Virgin Islands

Virgin Islands Medical
  Institute, Inc.
1AD Estate Diamond Ruby
P.O. Box 5989
Christiansted, St. Croix, VI
  00823-5989
809-778-6470

SECTION D

Insurance Departments

Alabama

Insurance Department
Retirement Systems Building
201 Monroe, Suite 1700
Montgomery, AL 36104
Mail:
P.O. Box 303351
Montgomery, AL 36130-3351
334-269-3550

Alaska

Division of Insurance
Department of Commerce and
  Economic Development
State Office Building
333 Willoughby, 9th floor
Juneau, AK 99801
Mail:
P.O. Box 110805
Juneau, AK 99811-0805
907-465-2515
800-467-8725 (Alaska only)

Arizona

Insurance Department
2910 North 44th Street,
  Suite 210
Phoenix, AZ 85018-7256

602-912-8400
800-325-2548 (Arizona only)

Arkansas

Insurance Department
1200 West Third Street
Little Rock, AR 72201-1904
501-371-2600
800-282-9134

California

Department of Insurance
300 South Spring Street
Los Angeles, CA 90013
213-897-8921

Colorado

Division of Insurance
1560 Broadway, Suite 850
Denver, CO 80202
303-894-7499

Connecticut

Insurance Department
P.O. Box 816
Hartford, CT 06142-0816
860-297-3800
800-203-3447

Delaware

Insurance Department
First Federal Plaza
710 North King Street,
  Suite 350
Wilmington, DE 19801
302-577-3119
800-282-8611

District of Columbia

Insurance Administration
Department of Insurance
  and Security Regulations
441 4th Street NW, Suite 870
  North
Washington, DC 20001
202-727-7424

Florida

Department of Insurance
Insurance Consumer Services
  Division
Larson Building
200 East Gaines Street
Tallahassee, FL 32399-0300
904-922-3100
800-342-2762 (Florida only)

Georgia

Office of Commissioner
  of Insurance
Floyd Memorial Building,
  West Tower, 9th Floor
2 Martin Luther King, Jr.
  Drive
Atlanta, GA 30334
404-656-2056

800-656-2298 (Georgia only)
404-656-4031 (TDD)

Hawaii

Insurance Division
Department of Commerce
  and Consumer Affairs
P.O. Box 3614
Honolulu, HI 96811-3614
808-586-2790

Idaho

Idaho Department of Insurance
700 West State, 3rd Floor
P.O. Box 83720
Boise, ID 83720-0043
208-334-4350
800-247-4422 (Boise only)
800-488-5728 (Lewiston only)
800-488-5764 (Pocatello only)
800-488-5731 (Twin Falls only)

Illinois

Department of Insurance
320 West Washington Street
Springfield, IL 62767
217-782-4515
217-524-4872 (TDD)

Indiana

Department of Insurance
311 West Washington Street,
  Suite 300
Indianapolis, IN 46204
317-232-2385
800-622-4461 (Indiana only)

Iowa

Division of Insurance
Department of Commerce
Lucas State Office Building
Des Moines, IA 50319
515-281-5705

Kansas

Insurance Department
420 SW 9th Street
Topeka, KS 66612-1678
913-296-3071
800-432-2484 (Kansas only)

Kentucky

Department of Insurance
Public Protection and
  Regulation Cabinet
Sullivan Building
215 West Main Street
Frankfort, KY 40601
502-564-3630
800-595-6053 (Kentucky
  only)
800-462-2081 (TDD)

Louisiana

Insurance Building
P.O. Box 94214
Baton Rouge, LA 70804-9214
504-342-5900
800-259-5300 (Louisiana
  only)

Maine

Bureau of Insurance
Department of Professional
  and Financial Regulation
124 Northern Avenue
Gardner, ME 04345
Mail:
Bureau of Insurance
Department of Professional
  and Financial Regulation
34 State House Station
Augusta, ME 04333
207-624-8475
800-300-5000 (Maine only)
207-624-8563 (TDD)

Maryland

Insurance Administration
525 St. Paul Place
Baltimore, MD 21202
410-468-2000
800-492-6116
800-552-7724 (TDD)

Massachusetts

Division of Insurance
470 Atlantic Avenue, 6th Floor
Boston, MA 02210
617-521-7794
617-521-7490 (TDD)

Michigan

Insurance Bureau
P.O. Box 30220
Lansing, MI 48909-7720
517-373-9273

Minnesota

Insurance Division
Department of Commerce
133 East 7th Street
St. Paul, MN 55101
612-296-4026
800-657-3602 (Minnesota
  only)
612-296-2860 (TDD)

Mississippi

Insurance Department
550 High Street, Suite 1804
Jackson, MS 39201
Mail:
P.O. Box 79
Jackson, MS 39205
601-359-3569
800-562-2957

Missouri

Division of Insurance
301 West High Street,
  Suite 630
P.O. Box 690
Jefferson City, MO 65102-
  0690
573-751-2640
800-726-7390
573-526-4536 (TDD)

Montana

Commissioner of Insurance
State Auditor Office
P.O. Box 4009
Helena, MT 59604-4009
406-444-2040

800-332-6148 (Montana
  only)
406-444-3246 (TDD)

Nebraska

Department of Insurance
941 O Street, Suite 400
Lincoln, NE 68508
402-471-2201
800-833-7352 (TDD)

Nevada

Department of Business
  and Industry
Insurance Division
1665 Hot Springs Road,
  Room 152
Carson City, NV 89706
702-687-4270
800-992-0900 x4270
  (Nevada only)

New Hampshire

Insurance Department
169 Manchester Street
Concord, NH 03301-5151
603-271-2261
800-852-3416 (New
  Hampshire only)
800-735-2964 (TDD)

New Jersey

Department of Insurance
20 West State Street
P.O. Box 329
Trenton, NJ 08625-0329
609-292-5360

New Mexico

Department of Insurance
State Corporation
  Commission
Pera Building, P.O. Drawer
  1269
Santa Fe, NM 87504-1269
505-827-4601
800-947-4722 (New Mexico
  only)

New York

Insurance Department
25 Beaver Street
New York, NY 10004
212-480-6400
800-342-3736
800-220-9250 (TDD)

North Carolina

Department of Insurance
401 Glenwood Avenue
Raleigh, NC 27603
919-733-2205

North Dakota

Insurance Department
State Capitol, 5th Floor
600 East Boulevard Avenue
Bismarck, ND 58505-0320
701-328-2440
800-247-0560 (North
  Dakota only)
800-366-6888 (TTY)

Ohio

Department of Insurance
2100 Stella Court
Columbus, OH 43215-1067
614-644-2658
800-686-1526
800-750-0750 (TDD)

Oklahoma

Insurance Department
P.O. Box 53408
Oklahoma City, OK 73152-
  3408
405-521-6628
800-763-2828 (Oklahoma
  only)

Oregon

Department of Consumer
  and Business Services
Insurance Division
Consumer Services and
  Enforcement
350 Winter Street NE,
  Room 440-2
Salem, OR 97310
503-947-7980 (also TDD)
800-722-4134

Pennsylvania

Department of Insurance
1321 Strawberry Square
Harrisburg, PA 17120
717-787-2317
717-783-3898 (TDD)

Rhode Island

Department of Business
and Regulation
Office of the Commissioner
Insurance Division
233 Richmond Street,
Suite 233
Providence, RI 02903-4233
401-222-2223 (also TDD)

South Carolina

Office of the Commissioner
Department of Insurance
1612 Marion Street
Columbia, SC 29201
803-737-6227
800-768-3467

South Dakota

Division of Insurance
Department of Commerce
and Regulation
118 West Capitol
Pierre, SD 57501-2000
605-773-4104

Tennessee

Department of Commerce
and Insurance
500 James Robertson
Parkway
Nashville, TN 37243-0565
615-741-2241
615-741-0481 (TDD)

Texas

Texas Department of
Insurance
Consumer Protection
Division
333 Guadalupe Street,
MC 111-1A
Austin, TX 78701
Mail:
P.O. Box 149091
Austin, TX 78714-9091
512-463-6515
800-252-3439
512-322-4238 (TDD)

Utah

Insurance Department
State Office Building,
Room 3110
Salt Lake City, UT 84114
www.ins-dept.state.ut.us
801-538-3800
800-439-3805
801-538-3826 (TDD)

Vermont

Banking, Insurance and
Securities
89 Main Street, Drawer 20
Montpelier, VT 05620-3101
802-828-3301

Virginia

Bureau of Insurance
1300 E. Main Street
Richmond, VA 23219
Mail:
P.O. Box 1157
Richmond, VA 23218
804-371-9741
800-552-7945 (Virginia only)
804-371-9206 (TDD)

Washington

Office of the Insurance
  Commissioner
Insurance Building
P.O. Box 40256
Olympia, WA 98504-0256
360-407-0383
800-397-4422 (Washington
  only)

West Virginia

Department of Insurance
1124 Smith Street
Charleston, WV 25301
Mail:
P.O. Box 50540
Charleston, WV 25305-0540
304-558-3386
800-642-9004 (West Virginia
  only)

Wisconsin

Office of the Commissioner
  of Insurance
121 East Wilson
Madison, WI 53702

Mail:
P.O. Box 7873
Madison, WI 53707-7873
608-266-3585
800-236-8517 (Wisconsin
  only)
800-947-3529 (TDD)

Wyoming

Insurance Department
Herschler Building, 3rd
  Floor East
122 West 25th Street
Cheyenne, WY 82002
307-777-7401
800-438-5768 (Wyoming
  only)

Puerto Rico

Office of the Insurance
  Commissioner
P.O. Box 8330
Fernandez Juncos Station
Santurce, PR 00910-8330
787-722-8686

Virgin Islands

Office of the Lieutenant
  Governor
Lieutenant Governor's
  Office Building
18 Kongens Gade
St. Thomas, VI 00802
340-774-2991

State Medicaid Offices

Alabama
Medicaid Agency
501 Dexter Avenue
P.O. Box 5624
Montgomery, AL 36103-5624
334-242-5000
334-242-5010 (TDD)

Alaska
Department of Health
  and Social Services
Division of Medical
  Assistance
P.O. Box 110660
Juneau, AK 99811-0660
907-465-3355 (also TDD)

Arizona
Arizona Health Care Cost
  Containment System
801 East Jefferson Street
Phoenix, AZ 85034
602-417-4000
800-654-8713 (Arizona only)

Arkansas
Department of Human
  Services
Division of Medical Services

P.O. Box 1437, Slot 1100
Little Rock, AR 72203-1437
501-682-8292
501-682-7958 (TDD)

California
Department of Health
  Services
714 P Street, Room 1253
Sacramento, CA 95814
916-657-1425

Colorado
Department of Health Care
  Policy and Financing
1575 Sherman Street,
  4th Floor
Denver, CO 80203-1714
303-866-6092
303-866-3833 (TTY)

Connecticut
Department of Social
  Services
25 Sigourney Street
Hartford, CT 06106
860-424-4925
800-443-9946

Delaware
Department of Health
  and Social Services
1901 North Du Pont
  Highway
P.O. Box 906
New Castle, DE 19720
302-577-4901
800-372-2022 (Delware
  only)
800-924-3958 (TDD)

District of Columbia
Commission on Health
  Care Finance
2100 Martin Luther
  King, Jr. Avenue SE
Suite 302
Washington, DC 20020
202-727-0735

Florida
Agency for Health Care
  Administration
2728 Mahan Drive,
  Suite 2417
Tallahassee, FL 32308
Mail:
Agency for Health Care
  Administration
P.O. Box 13000
Tallahassee, FL 32317-
  3000
904-488-3560

Georgia
Department of Medical
  Assistance
2 Peachtree Street NW
40th Floor, Suite 4043
Atlanta, GA 30303-3159
404-656-4479
800-869-1150

Hawaii
Department of Human
  Services
Med Quest Division
P.O. Box 339
Honolulu, HI 96809-0339
808-586-5391
808-587-3520 (TDD)

Idaho
Department of Health
  and Welfare
Towers Building, 3rd Floor
P.O. Box 83720
Boise, ID 83720-0036
208-334-5747

Illinois
Department of Public Aid
Division of Medical
  Programs
201 South Grand Avenue
  East
3rd Floor
Springfield, IL 62763-0001
217-782-2570

Indiana

Medicaid Policy and Planning
Family and Social Services
 Administration
402 West Washington Street,
 Room W382
P.O. Box 7083
Indianapolis, IN 46207-7083
317-233-4455
800-457-4584
800-962-8408 (TDD)

Iowa

Department of Human
 Services
Division of Medical Services
Hoover State Office Building,
 5th Floor
1305 E. Walnut
Des Moines, IA 50319-0114
515-281-8621 (accepts collect
 calls)

Kansas

Department of Social and
 Rehabilitative Services
Docking State Office
 Building, 628 South
Topeka, KS 66612
913-296-3981

Kentucky

Department of Medicaid
 Services
275 East Main Street, 6 W-A
Frankfort, KY 40621
502-564-4321

Louisiana

Department of Health and
 Hospitals
1201 Capitol Access Road
Baton Rouge, LA 70801
Mail:
Department of Health and
 Hospitals
P.O. Box 91030
Baton Rouge, LA 70821-9030
504-342-3891

Maine

Department of Human
 Services
Bureau of Medical Services
State House Station 11
Augusta, ME 04333
207-287-2674
800-321-5557

Maryland

Department of Health and
 Mental Hygiene
Herbert R. O'Conor Building
201 West Preston Street,
 5th Floor
Baltimore, MD 21201
410-767-6505
800-735-2258 (TTY)

Massachusetts

Division of Medical Assistance
600 Washington Street
Boston, MA 02111
617-210-5690
800-841-2900

Michigan

Medical Services
  Administration
Department of
  Community Health
P.O. Box 30479
Lansing, MI 48909
517-335-5001
800-638-6414

Minnesota

Health Care Administration
Department of Human Services
444 Lafayette Road, 6th Floor
St. Paul, MN 55155-3852
612-296-3386
800-657-3756
800-657-3729

Mississippi

Division of Medicaid
Office of the Governor
Robert E. Lee Building
239 North Lamar Street,
  Suite 801
Jackson, MS 39201-1399
601-359-6050
800-421-2408

Missouri

Department of Social Services
Division of Medical Services
615 Howerton Court
P.O. Box 6500
Jefferson City, MO 65102-
  6500
573-751-3425

Montana

Department of Public Health
  and Human Services
1400 Broadway
P.O. Box 202951
Helena, MT 59620
406-444-4540

Nebraska

Nebraska Health and
  Human Services System
Medical Services Division
301 Centennial Mall South,
  5th Floor
P.O. Box 95026
Lincoln, NE 68509-5026
402-471-3121
800-833-7352 (also TDD)

Nevada

Department of Human
  Resources
Welfare Division
2527 North Carson Street
Carson City, NV 89710
702-687-4770

New Hampshire

Health and Human Services
Office of Health Management
Medicaid Administration
  Bureau
6 Hazen Drive
Concord, NH 03301-6521
603-271-4353
800-852-3345
800-735-2964 (TDD)

New Jersey

Human Services Department
Medical Assistance and
  Health Services Division
7 Quakerbridge Plaza
P.O. Box 712
Trenton, NJ 08625
609-588-2600

New Mexico

Department of Human
  Services
Medical Assistance Division
P.O. Box 2348
Santa Fe, NM 87504-2348
505-827-3106
800-432-6217

New York

State Department of Health
Office of Medicaid Manage-
  ment
Corning Tower, Empire
  State Plaza
Albany, NY 12237
518-474-2482

North Carolina

Division of Medical
  Assistance
1985 Umstead Drive
P.O. Box 29529
Raleigh, NC 27626-0529
919-733-2060
800-662-7030

North Dakota

Department of Human Services
Medical Services
600 East Boulevard Avenue
Bismarck, ND 58505-0261
701-328-2321
800-755-2604 (North Dakota
  only)

Ohio

Department of Human Services
Office of Medicaid
30 East Broad Street, 31st Floor
Columbus, OH 43266-0423
614-644-0140
800-342-8680
614-752-3951 (TDD)

Oklahoma

Health Care Authority
4545 North Lincoln Boulevard,
  Suite 124
Oklahoma City, OK 73105
405-530-3439

Oregon

Department of Human
  Resources
Office of Medical Assistance
  Programs
500 Summer Street NE
Salem, OR 97310-1014
503-945-5772
800-527-5772
800-375-2863 (TDD)

Pennsylvania

Department of Public
  Welfare
Medical Assistance Programs
Health and Welfare Building,
  Room 515
P.O. Box 2675
Harrisburg, PA 17105-2675
717-787-1870
800-772-6142

Rhode Island

Department of Human
  Services
Division of Medical Services
600 New London Avenue
Cranston, RI 02920
401-464-2121

South Carolina

Department of Health
  and Human Services
P.O. Box 8206
Columbia, SC 29202-8206
803-253-6100

South Dakota

Department of Social Services
Medical Services Offices
Kneip Building
700 Governor's Drive
Pierre, SD 57501-2291
605-773-3495

Tennessee

Department of Health
Bureau of Tenncare
729 Church Street
Nashville, TN 37247
615-741-0213
800-342-3145
800-772-7647 (TDD)

Texas

Texas Department of Health
Health Care Financing
1100 West 49th Street
Austin, TX 78759
512-338-6500
800-252-8263 (also TDD)

Utah

Department of Health
Health Care Financing
Medicaid Information Unit
288 North 1460 West,
  3rd Floor
Salt Lake City, UT 84116-
  0580
801-538-6406
800-662-9651 (Utah only)

Vermont

Human Services Agency
Medicaid Division
103 South Main Street
Waterbury, VT 05671-1201
802-241-2880
800-987-2839 (Vermont
  only)

Virginia

Department of Medical
  Services
Division of Medical
  Social Services
600 East Broad Street,
  Suite 1300
Richmond, VA 23219
804-786-8099

Washington

Washington State Medical
  Assistance Administration
P.O. Box 45080
Olympia, WA 98504-5080
360-902-7806

West Virginia

Department of Health
  and Human Resources
Bureau for Medical Services
State Capitol Complex,
  Building 6
Charleston, WV 25305
304-926-1700
800-642-3607 (West
  Virginia only)

Wisconsin

Bureau of Health Care
  Financing
Department of Health
  and Family Services
Division of Health

1 West Wilson Street,
  Room 250
Madison, WI 53701
608-266-2522
608-221-5720 (Dane County
  only)
800-362-3002 (Wisconsin
  only)

Wyoming

Department of Health
Division of Health Care
  Financing
6101 Yellowstone Road
Cheyenne, WY 82002
307-777-7531
307-777-5648 (TTY)

Puerto Rico

Office of Economic Assis-
  tance to the Medically
  Indigent
GPO Box 70184
San Juan, PR 00936
787-765-1230

Virgin Islands

Bureau of Health Insurance
  and Medical Assistance
Health Department
Frostco Center, Suite 302
210-3A Altona
Charlotte Amalie, St.
  Thomas, VI 00802
809-774-4624

SECTION F

Long-Term Care Ombudsmen Offices

Alabama

Commission on Aging
770 Washington Avenue,
  Suite 470
Montgomery, AL 36130-1851
334-242-5743
800-243-5463

Alaska

Older Alaskans' Commission
Department of Administration
3601 C Street, Suite 260
Anchorage, AK 99503
907-563-6393
800-730-6393 (Alaska only)

Arizona

State Agency on Aging
Aging and Adult Admin-
  istration
1789 West Jefferson
Phoenix, AZ 85007
602-542-4446

Arkansas

Division of Aging and
  Adult Services
Department of Human
  Services
1417 Donaghey Plaza
  South
P.O. Box 1437, Slot 1412
Little Rock, AR 72203-1437
501-682-2441
501-682-2443 (TDD)

California

Department of Aging
Office of the Long Term
  Care Ombudsman
1600 K Street
Sacramento, CA 95814
916-322-5290
800-231-4024 (California
  only)
800-735-2929 (TDD)

Colorado

State Care Ombudsman
  Program
455 Sherman Street, Suite 130
Denver, CO 80203
303-722-0300 (also TDD)
800-288-1376 (Colorado
  only; also TDD)

Connecticut

Department of Social
  Services
Division of Elderly Services
25 Sigourney Street
Hartford, CT 06106
860-424-5200

Delaware (Northern)

Division of Aging & Adults
  with Physical Disabilities
Attn: LTCO
Oxford Bldg., Suite 200
256 Chapman Road
Newark, DE 19702
302-453-3820
800-273-9074

Delaware (Southern)

Division Aging and Adults
  with Physical Disabilities
Milford State Service Center
18 North Walnut Street
Milford, DE 19963
302-422-1386
800-273-9074
302-422-1415 (TDD)

District of Columbia

Legal Council for the Elderly
601 E Street NW
Washington, DC 20049
202-434-2140
202-434-6562 (TDD)

Florida

Long-Term Care Ombudsman
  Council
600 S. Calhoun Street,
  Suite 270
Tallahassee, FL 32301
904-488-6190

Georgia

Division of Aging Services
Department of Human
  Resources
2 Peachtree Street NW,
  36th Floor
Atlanta, GA 30303
404-657-5319

Hawaii

Executive Office on Aging
250 W. Hotel Street, Suite 109
Honolulu, HI 96813
808-586-0100
800-484-4454

Idaho

Office on Aging
State House
P.O. Box 83720
Boise, ID 83720-0007
208-334-4693

Illinois

Department on Aging
421 East Capitol Avenue,
    Suite 100
Springfield, IL 62701-1789
217-785-3143
800-252-8966 (also TDD)

Indiana

Bureau of Aging and
    In-Home Services
402 West Washington,
    Room W454
P.O. Box 7083
Indianapolis, IN 46207-7083
317-232-7134
800-622-4484
317-232-1143 (TDD)

Iowa

Department of Elder Affairs
Clemens Building, 3rd Floor
200 10th Street
Des Moines, IA 50309-3609
515-281-5426
800-532-3213 (Complaint
    Hotline)
515-281-5188 (TDD)

Kansas

Department on Aging
Docking State Office
    Building
915 SW Harrison Street,
    Room 150-S
Topeka, KS 66612-1500
913-296-4986

Kentucky

Department of Social
    Services
Division of Aging Services
CHR Building, 5W
275 East Main Street
Frankfort, KY 40621
502-564-6930
800-372-2991

Louisiana

Governor's Office of
    Elderly Affairs
Elder Rights
P.O. Box 80374
Baton Rouge, LA 70898-0374
504-342-7100
800-259-4990

Maine

Long-Term Care
    Ombudsman Program
P.O. Box 126
Augusta, ME 04332
207-621-1079
800-499-0229

Maryland

Office on Aging
301 West Preston Street,
    Room 1007
Baltimore, MD 21201
410-767-1100
800-243-3425
410-767-1083 (TDD)

Massachusetts

Elder Affairs Executive
  Offices
McCormack Building
One Ashburton Place, 5th
  Floor
Boston, MA 02108
617-727-7750
800-882-2003
800-872-0166 (TDD)

Michigan

Citizens for Better Care
4750 Woodward, Suite 410
Detroit, MI 48201-1308
313-832-6387
800-833-9548

Minnesota

Board on Aging
Human Services Building
444 Lafayette Road
St. Paul, MN 55155-3843
612-296-0382
800-296-2544

Mississippi

Council on Aging
750 N. State Street
Jackson, MS 39205
601-359-4929

Missouri

Department of Social Services
Aging Division
615 Howerton Court
P.O. Box 1337
Jefferson City, MO 65102
573-751-3082
800-309-3282

Montana

Office on Aging
Department of Public Health
  & Human Services
Capitol Station
P.O. Box 4210
Helena, MT 59604-4210
406-444-4676
800-332-2272 (Montana only)

Nebraska

Department on Aging
P.O. Box 95044
Lincoln, NE 68509-5044
402-471-2307
800-942-7830 (Nebraska only)
402-471-4619 (TDD)

Nevada

Aging Services Administration
Human Resources Depart-
  ment
340 North 11th Street, Suite
  203
Las Vegas, NV 89101
702-486-3545
800-677-1116

New Hampshire

Long-Term Care Ombudsman
6 Hazen Drive
Concord, NH 03301
603-271-4375
800-442-5640

New Jersey

Department of Health and
  Senior Services
Ombudsman for the Elderly
PO Box 807
Trenton, NJ 08625-0807
609-292-8016
800-792-8820 (New Jersey
  only)

New Mexico

State Agency on Aging
La Villa Rivera Building
228 East Palace Avenue
Santa Fe, NM 87501
505-827-7640
800-432-2080

New York

Office for Aging
2 Empire State Plaza
Albany, NY 12223
518-474-7329
800-342-9871

North Carolina

Division of Aging
693 Palmer Drive
Raleigh, NC 27626
919-733-3983

North Dakota

Long Term Care Ombudsman
Aging Services Division
600 South Second Street,
  Suite 1C
Bismarck, ND 58504-5729
701-328-8910
800-755-8521 (North Dakota
  only)
701-328-8968 (TDD)

Ohio

Department on Aging
State Ombudsman
50 West Broad Street, 9th
  Floor
Columbus, OH 43215
614-466-1221
800-282-1206
614-466-6191 (TDD)

Oklahoma

DHS – Aging Services Division
Long Term Care Ombudsman
312 NE 28th Street
Oklahoma City, OK 73105
405-521-6734

Oregon

Long-Term Care Ombudsman
3855 Wolverine NE, Suite 6
Salem, OR 97310
503-378-6533
800-522-2602 (Oregon only)
503-378-5847 (TDD)

Pennsylvania

Long-Term Care Ombudsman
Department of Aging
555 Walnut Street
Forum Place, 5th Floor
Harrisburg, PA 17101-1919
717-783-7247

Rhode Island

Department of Elderly Affairs
160 Pine Street
Providence, RI 02903
401-277-2858
800-322-2880 (Rhode
  Island only)

South Carolina

Department of Health and
  Human Services
Division on Aging
1801 Main Street
Columbia, SC 29202-8206
803-253-6177
800-868-9095 (SC only)

South Dakota

Office of Adult Services
  and Aging
Social Services Department
700 Governor's Drive
Pierre, SD 57501-2291
605-773-3656

Tennessee

Commission on Aging
500 Deaderick Street,
  9th Floor
Nashville, TN 37243-0860
615-741-2056

Texas

Department on Aging
Nursing Home Advocacy
  and Long-Term Care
  Ombudsman
P.O. Box 12786
Austin, TX 78711
512-424-6840
800-252-2412

Utah

Long-Term Care Ombudsman
120 North 200 West,
  Room 325
Salt Lake City, UT 84103
801-538-3910

Vermont

Long Term Care Ombudsman
  Program
264 N. Winooski Avenue
Burlington, VT 05402
802-863-5620 (also TTY)
800-747-5022 (Vermont
  only; also TTY)

Virginia

State Long Term Care
   Ombudsman
Virginia Association of
   Agencies on Aging
530 East Main Street,
   Suite 428
Richmond, VA 23219
804-644-2804
800-552-3402 (Virginia only)

Washington

Long-Term Care Ombudsman
Aging and Adult Services
   Administration
600 Woodland Square Loop
   SE, Bldg. A
P.O. Box 45600
Olympia, WA 98504-5600
206-493-2560
800-422-3263
360-493-2637 (TTY)

West Virginia

Bureau of Senior Services
State Capitol Complex
1900 Kanawha Boulevard East
Holly Grove, Bldg. 10
Charleston, WV 25305-0160
304-558-3317

Wisconsin

Board on Aging
214 North Hamilton Street
Madison, WI 53703-2118
608-266-8944 (also TDD)
800-242-1060 (Wisconsin
   only)

Wyoming

Long-Term Care Ombudsman
P.O. Box 94
Wheatland, WY 82201
307-322-5553

Puerto Rico

Office of the Ombudsman
Manillas Station
P.O. Box 41088
San Juan, PR 00940-1088
787-724-7373

Aging Agencies

Alabama

Commission on Aging
770 Washington Avenue,
  Suite 470
Montgomery, AL 36130-1851
334-242-5743
800-243-5463

Alaska

Alaskan Commission on Aging
P.O. Box 110209
Juneau, AK 99811-0209
907-465-3250
800-478-6065 (Alaska only)
907-465-3650 (Insurance
  counseling)
800-478-6065 (Medicare
  Hotline)

Arizona

Economic Security Department
Division of Aging and
  Community Services
1789 West Jefferson, 001A
Phoenix, AZ 85007
602-542-4446
602-542-6572
602-542-6446 (insurance
  counseling)

Arkansas

Human Services Department
Division of Aging and Adult
  Services
1417 Donaghey Building
  Plaza South
P.O. Box 1437, Slot 1412
Little Rock, AR 72203-1437
501-682-2441
501-371-2782 (insurance
  counseling)
800-852-5494 (insurance
  counseling)
501-682-2443 (TDD)

California

Department of Aging
1600 K Street
Sacramento, CA 95814
916-322-3887
916-323-7315 (insurance
  counseling)
800-510-2020 (California
  only)
800-735-2929 (TDD)

Colorado

Commission on Aging
Aging and Adult Services
110 16th Street, Suite 200
Denver, CO 80202
303-620-4146
303-899-5151 (insurance
counseling)
800-544-9181 (insurance
counseling Colorado only)

Connecticut

Department of Social Services
Elderly Services Division
25 Sigourney Street,
10th Floor
Hartford, CT 06106
860-424-4925
800-443-9946 (Connecticut
only)
800-994-9422 (insurance
counseling Connecticut
only)

Delaware

Health and Social Services
Department
Aging Division
1901 North DuPont
Highway
New Castle, DE 19720
302-577-4660
800-223-9074 (Delaware
only)
800-282-8611
800-336-9500 (insurance
counseling)

District of Columbia

Aging Office
1 Judiciary Square
441 4th Street NW,
Suite 900 South
Washington, DC 20001
202-724-5622
202-676-3900 (insurance
counseling)

Florida

Department of Elder Affairs
4040 Esplanade Way
Building B, Suite 152
Tallahassee, FL 32399-7000
904-414-2000
904-414-2060 (insurance
counseling)
904-414-2001 (TDD)

Georgia

Human Resources Department
Division of Aging Services
2 Peachtree Street NW,
Suite 36-385
Atlanta, GA 30303
404-657-5258
800-669-8387 (insurance
counseling)

Hawaii

Executive Office on Aging
250 South Hotel Street, Suite 109
Honolulu, HI 96813
808-586-0100
808-586-7299 (insurance
counseling)

Idaho

Commission on Aging
700 West Jefferson, Room 108
Boise, ID 83702
208-334-3833
208-334-4350 (insurance
  counseling)
800-247-4422 (insurance
  counseling)
800-377-3529 (TDD)

Illinois

Department on Aging
421 East Capitol Avenue, #100
Springfield, IL 62701-1789
217-785-3356
800-252-8966 (Illinois only,
  TTY, insurance counseling)

Indiana

Family and Social Services
  Administration
Bureau of Aging Services
402 West Washington Street
Indianapolis, IN 46207-7083
317-232-7020
800-545-7763 (Indiana only)

Iowa

Elder Affairs Department
Clemens Bldg, 3rd Floor
200 10th Street
Des Moines, IA 50309
515-281-5187
800-351-4664 (insurance
  counseling)

Kansas

Department on Aging
150-S Docking State Office
  Building
915 SW Harrison
Topeka, KS 66612-1500
913-296-4986 (also TDD)
800-432-3535 (Kansas only)
800-860-5260 (insurance
  counseling)

Kentucky

Department of Social Services
Aging Services Division
275 East Main Street
Frankfort, KY 40621-0001
502-564-6930

Louisiana

Office of Elderly Affairs
P.O. Box 80374
Baton Rouge, LA 70898-0374
504-342-7100
504-342-5301 (insurance
  counseling)
800-259-5301 (insurance
  counseling)

Maine

Human Services Department
Elder and Adult Services
  Bureau
State House Station 11
35 Anthony Avenue
Augusta, ME 04333-0011
207-624-5335 (insurance
  counseling)

Maryland

Office on Aging
301 West Preston Street,
  Room 1007
Baltimore, MD 21201
410-767-1100
800-243-3425

Massachusetts

Elder Affairs Executive Office
McCormack Building
One Ashburton Place,
  5th Floor
Boston, MA 02108
617-727-7750
800-882-2003 (also insurance
  counseling)
800-872-0166 (TDD)

Michigan

Office of Services to the
  Aging
611 West Ottawa Street,
  3rd Floor
P.O. Box 30676
Lansing, MI 48909-8176
517-373-8230
800-803-7176 (insurance
  counseling)
517-373-4096 (TDD)

Minnesota

Minnesota Board on Aging
Aging and Adult Services
  Division
Human Services Building
444 Lafayette Road

St. Paul, MN 55155-3843
612-296-2544
800-882-6262 (insurance
  counseling)

Mississippi

Human Services Department
Division of Aging and Adult
  Services
750 N. State Street
Jackson, MS 39202
601-359-4929 (also insurance
  counseling)
800-948-3090 (also insurance
  counseling)

Missouri

Social Services Department
Division of Aging
615 Howerton Court
Jefferson City, MO 65109
Mail:
P.O. Box 1337
Jefferson City, MO 65102
573-751-3082
800-390-3330 (insurance
  counseling)

Montana

Senior and Long-Term Care
  Division
Department on Aging
P.O. Box 4210
Helena, MT 59620
406-444-4077
800-332-2272 (insurance
  counseling)

271

Nebraska

Department on Aging
301 Centennial Mall South
P.O. Box 95044
Lincoln, NE 68509-5044
402-471-2307
800-942-7830
402-471-2307 (insurance
counseling)
402-471-2306 (TDD)

Nevada

Human Resources Department
Aging Services
505 East King Street,
Room 600
Carson City, NV 89710
702-486-3545

New Hampshire

Health and Human Services
Department
Elderly and Adult Services
Division
Office Park South
115 Pleasant Street, Annex #1
Concord, NH 03301-3843
603-271-4680
800-351-1888 (New Hampshire
only)
800-852-3388 (insurance
counseling)

New Jersey

Department of Health and
Senior Services

Division of Senior Affairs
CN 807
101 South Broad and Front
Streets
Trenton, NJ 08625-0807
609-984-6693
800-792-8820 (New Jersey
only)

New Mexico

State Agency on Aging
La Villa Rivera Building
228 East Palace Avenue
Santa Fe, NM 87501
505-827-7640
800-432-2080 (New Mexico
only)

New York

Office for Aging
2 Empire State Plaza
Albany, NY 12223-1251
518-474-8675
800-342-9871 (insurance
counseling, NY only)
518-474-0608 (TTY)

North Carolina

Department of Health
and Human Services
Division of Aging
693 Palmer Drive
CB29531
Raleigh, NC 27626-0531
919-733-3983
800-443-9354 (insurance
counseling)

North Dakota

Human Services Department
Aging Services Division
State Capitol-Judicial Wing
600 South Second Street,
  Suite 1C
Bismarck, ND 58504-5729
701-328-8910
800-755-8521 (North Dakota
  only)
701-328-8968 (TDD)
701-328-2440 (insurance
  counseling)

Ohio

Department on Aging
50 West Broad Street,
  8th Floor
Columbus, OH 43215-5928
614-466-5500
614-466-6191 (TDD)
800-686-1578 (insurance
  counseling)

Oklahoma

Department of Human
  Services
Aging Services Division
312 NE 28th Street
Oklahoma City, OK 73125
Mail:
P.O. Box 25352
Oklahoma City, OK 73125
405-521-2327
800-763-2828 (insurance
  counseling)

Oregon

Human Resources
  Department
Senior and Disabled Services
  Division
Human Resources Building
500 Summer Street NE
Salem, OR 97310-1015
503-945-5811 (also TTY)
800-282-8096 (Oregon only)
800-722-4134 (insurance
  counseling)

Pennsylvania

Department of Aging
555 Walnut Street, 5th Floor
Harrisburg, PA 17101-1919
717-783-1550
800-783-7067 (insurance
  counseling)

Rhode Island

Department of Elderly Affairs
160 Pine Street
Providence, RI 02903
401-222-2858 (insurance
  counseling)
800-322-2880 (TDD and
  Rhode Island only)

South Carolina

Department of Health and
Human Services
Office on Aging
1801 Main Street
P.O. Box 8206
Columbia, SC 29202-8206
803-253-6177
800-868-9095 (insurance
counseling and South
Carolina only)

South Dakota

Social Services Department
Adult Services and Aging Office
700 Governor's Drive
Pierre, SD 57501-2291
605-773-3656 (also insurance
counseling)

Tennessee

Commission on Aging
500 Deaderick Street
Andrew Jackson Bldg. 9th Floor
Nashville, TN 37243-0860
615-741-2056
615-741-2241 (insurance
counseling)

Texas

Department on Aging
4900 North Lamar Boulevard
Austin, TX 78751
512-424-6840
800-332-0913 (insurance
counseling)

Utah

Human Services Department
Aging and Adult Services
120 North 200 West
P.O. Box 45500
Salt Lake City, UT 84103-0500
801-538-3910 (also insurance
counseling)

Vermont

Human Services Agency
Aging and Disabilities
Department
State Complex
103 South Main Street
Waterbury, VT 05671-2301
802-241-2400 (also TDD)
802-642-5199 (insurance
counseling)

Virginia

Department for the Aging
16 Forest Avenue, Suite 102
Richmond, VA 23229
804-662-9333 (also TDD)
800-552-3402 (insurance counseling and Virginia only)

Washington

Aging and Adult Services
Administration
P.O. Box 45600
Olympia, WA 98504-5600
360-493-2509 (insurance
counseling)
800-422-3263

West Virginia

Bureau of Senior Services
Holly Grove-State Capitol
  Complex
1900 Kanawha Boulevard
  East
Charleston, WV 25305
304-558-3317 (also insurance
  counseling)

Wisconsin

Department of Health and
  Family Service
Division of Supported Living
Bureau on Aging
217 S. Hamilton, Suite 300
Madison, WI 53703
608-266-2536 (also insurance
  counseling)

Wyoming

Health Department
Division on Aging
139 Hathaway Building
Cheyenne, WY 82002
307-777-7986
800-442-2766

Puerto Rico

Governor's Office on
  Elderly Affairs
P.O. Box 50063
Old San Juan Station
San Juan, PR 00902
787-721-4560

Virgin Islands

Department of Human
  Services
3011 Golden Rock
Christiansted, St. Croix,
  VI 00820
340-773-2980
340-773-2323, x101

State Attorney General Offices

Alabama

Attorney General
State House
111 South Union Street
Montgomery, AL 36130
334-242-7300

Alaska

Attorney General's Office
Department of Law
P.O. Box 110300
Juneau, AK 99811
907-465-3600

Arizona

Attorney General
1275 West Washington
Phoenix, AZ 85007
602-542-5025

Arkansas

Office of the Attorney General
200 Catlett-Prinn Tower
  Building
323 Center Street
Little Rock, AR 72201
501-682-2007
800-482-8982
501-682-6073 (TTY)

California

Office of the Attorney General
Department of Justice
P.O. Box 944255
Sacramento, CA 94244-2550
916-445-9555

Colorado

Attorney General
1525 Sherman Street, 5th Floor
Denver, CO 80203
303-866-3617

Connecticut

Attorney General
55 Elm Street
P.O. Box 120
Hartford, CT 06141-0120
860-808-5318

Delaware

Attorney General
Carvel State Office Building
820 North French Street
Wilmington, DE 19801
302-577-8400

District of Columbia

Honorable Janet Reno
Attorney General of the
  United States
Department of Justice
950 Pennsylvania Avenue
  NW, Room 4400
Washington, DC 20530-0001
202-514-2000

Florida

Attorney General
Department of Legal Affairs
PL-01 The Capitol
Tallahassee, FL 32399-1050
904-488-2526

Georgia

Attorney General
40 Capitol Square SW
Atlanta, GA 30334-1300
404-656-3300

Hawaii

Attorney General
425 Queen Street
Honolulu, HI 96813
808-586-1500

Idaho

Office of the Attorney
  General
210 Statehouse
P.O. Box 83720
Boise, ID 83720-0010
208-334-2400

Illinois

Attorney General
500 South Second Street
Springfield, IL 62706
217-782-1090
800-243-0618 (Central only)
217-785-2771 (TDD)
Second office location:
100 West Randolph, Suite 12
Chicago, IL 60601
312-814-3000
800-386-5438
312-814-3374 (TDD)

Indiana

Attorney General
402 West Washington Street,
  5th Floor
Indianapolis, IN 46204
317-232-6201
800-382-5516 (consumer
  protection and Indiana only)

Iowa

Attorney General
Hoover Building, 2nd Floor
Des Moines, IA 50319
515-281-5164

Kansas

Attorney General
Kansas Judicial Center,
  2nd Floor
Topeka, KS 66612
913-296-2215
800-432-2310 (Kansas only)
913-291-3767 (TDD)

Kentucky

Attorney General
State Capitol
1024 Capital Center Drive
Frankfort, KY 40601
502-696-5300

Louisiana

Attorney General
Department of Justice
P.O. Box 94005
Baton Rouge, LA 70804
504-342-7013

Maine

Attorney General
6 State House Station
Augusta, ME 04333
207-626-8800
207-626-8865 (TDD)

Maryland

Attorney General
200 Saint Paul Place
Baltimore, MD 21202
410-576-6300
410-576-6372 (TDD)

Massachusetts

Attorney General
One Ashburton Place,
  Room 2010
Boston, MA 02108
617-727-2200
617-727-0434 (TDD)

Michigan

Attorney General
G. Mennen Williams
  Building
P.O. Box 30212
Lansing, MI 48909
517-373-1110
517-373-1111 (TDD)

Minnesota

Attorney General
102 State Capitol
St. Paul, MN 55155
612-296-6196
800-657-3787 (consumer
  protection and Minnesota
  only)
612-297-7206 (TDD)
800-366-4812 (TDD)

Mississippi

Attorney General
P.O. Box 220
Jackson, MS 39205
601-359-3680
601-359-4231
800-281-4418 (Mississippi
  only)

Missouri

Attorney General Office
Supreme Court Building
P.O. Box 899
Jefferson City, MO 65102
573-751-3321
800-392-8222 (TDD and
  consumer protection)

Montana

Attorney General
Department of Justice
215 North Sanders
Helena, MT 59620
406-444-2026

Nebraska

Attorney General
2115 State Capitol
P.O. Box 98920
Lincoln, NE 68509
402-471-2682 (also TDD)

Nevada

Attorney General's Office
Capitol Complex
100 North Carson Street
Carson City, NV 89710
702-687-4170
800-992-0900 (Nevada only)
702-687-1382 (TDD)

New Hampshire

Attorney General
33 Capitol Street
Concord, NH 03301-6397
603-271-3658

New Jersey

Attorney General's Office
Department of Law and
   Public Safety
Justice Complex
P.O. Box 081
Trenton, NJ 08625-0081
609-984-1548

New Mexico

Attorney General
P.O. Drawer 1508
Santa Fe, NM 87504
505-827-6000

New York

Attorney General
Department of Law
State Capitol
Albany, NY 12224
518-474-7330

North Carolina

Attorney General
Department of Justice
P.O. Box 629
Raleigh, NC 27602
919-716-6400

North Dakota

Attorney General
State Capitol, 1st Floor
600 East Boulevard Avenue
Bismark, ND 58505
701-328-2210
800-472-2600 (consumer
   protection and ND only)
701-328-3409 (TDD)

Ohio

Attorney General
30 East Broad Street, 17th Floor
Columbus, OH 43215-3428
614-466-4320
800-282-0515 (consumer
   protection and Ohio only)

Oklahoma

Attorney General
2300 North Lincoln,
  Suite 112
Oklahoma City, OK 73105
405-521-3921

Oregon

Attorney General
1162 Court Street NE
Salem, OR 97310
503-378-4400
503-378-5938 (TDD)

Pennsylvania

Attorney General
Strawberry Square, 16th
  Floor
Harrisburg, PA 17120
717-787-3391
800-441-2555 (Consumer
  protection and PA only)

Rhode Island

Attorney General
150 South Main Street
Providence, RI 02903
401-274-4400
800-852-7776 (Consumer
  protection and Rhode
  Island)
401-453-0410 (TDD)

South Carolina

Attorney General
1000 Assembly Street,
  Suite 501
Columbia, SC 29202
Mail:
P.O. Box 11549
Columbia, SC 29211
803-734-3970

South Dakota

Attorney General
State Capitol
500 East Capitol Avenue
Pierre, SD 57501
605-773-3215
800-300-1986 (South
  Dakota only)
605-773-6585 (TDD)

Tennessee

Attorney General
415 Fifth Avenue North
Nashville, TN 37243-0497
615-741-3491

Texas

Attorney General
300 West 15th, 9th Floor
Austin, TX 78701
512-463-2185
800-252-8100

Utah
Attorney General
236 State Capitol
Salt Lake City, UT 84114
801-366-0260
800-244-4636 (Utah only)

Vermont
Attorney General
109 State Street
Montpelier, VT 05609
802-828-3171 (also TDD)

Virginia
Attorney General
900 East Main Street
Richmond, VA 23219
804-786-2071
800-752-8445 (TDD)

Washington
Attorney General
P.O. Box 40100
Olympia, WA 98504-0100
360-753-6200
800-551-4636 (Washington only)

West Virginia
Attorney General
State Capitol East Wing,
  Room 26
Charleston, WV 25305-0220
304-558-2021
800-368-8808

Wisconsin
Attorney General
Department of Justice
P.O. Box 7857
Madison, WI 53707
608-266-1221
608-267-8902 (TDD)

Wyoming
Attorney General
123 State Capitol
Cheyenne, WY 82002
307-777-7841
800-438-5799
307-777-5351 (TDD)

Puerto Rico
Attorney General's Office
Department of Justice
PO. Box 902192
San Juan, PR 00902-0192
787-721-7700

Virgin Islands
Attorney General
Department of Justice
48B-50C
Kronprindsens Gade,
  GERS Complex,
  2nd Floor
St. Thomas, VI 00802
340-774-5666

HCFA Regional Offices

Boston, Massachusetts

(serving Connecticut, Maine, Massachusetts, New Hampshire, Rhode Island, Vermont)
HCFA
J.F. Kennedy Bldg.,
  Room 2375
Boston, MA 02203
617-565-1232

New York, New York

(serving New York, New Jersey, Puerto Rico, Virgin Islands)
Division of Medicare
26 Federal Plaza
New York, NY 10278
212-264-3657

Philadelphia, Pennsylvania

(serving Delaware, District of Columbia, Maryland, Pennsylvania, Virginia, West Virginia)
HCFA
Region 3
3535 Market Street, 3rd Floor
Philadelphia, PA 19104
215-596-1335

Atlanta, Georgia

(serving Alabama, Florida, Georgia, Kentucky, Mississippi, North Carolina, South Carolina, Tennessee)
HCFA
101 Marietta Tower,
  Suite 702
Atlanta, GA 30323
404-331-2044
404-331-0108 (TDD)

Chicago, Illinois

(serving Illinois, Indiana, Michigan, Minnesota, Ohio, Wisconsin)
HCFA
105 West Adams
Chicago, IL 60603
312-353-7180

Dallas, Texas

(serving Arizona, Louisiana, New Mexico, Oklahoma, Texas)
HCFA
1301 Young Street, Room 827
Dallas, TX 75202
214-767-6401

Kansas City, Kansas

(serving Iowa, Kansas, Missouri, Nebraska)
HCFA
601 East 12th Street,
    Room 242
Kansas City, KS 64106
816-426-2866

Denver, Colorado

(serving Colorado, Montana, North Dakota, South Dakota, Utah)
Department of Health and
    Human Services Regional
    Office
Federal Office Building
Denver, CO 80294
303-844-4024

San Francisco, California

(serving Arizona, California, Guam, Hawaii, Nevada)
HCFA
75 Hawthorne Street,
    4th Floor
San Francisco, CA 94105
415-744-3602
415-744-3761

Seattle, Washington

(serving Alaska, Idaho, Oregon, Washington)
HCFA
2201 Sixth Avenue, RX-40
Seattle, WA 98121-2500
206-615-2306

SECTION J

Health Insurance Information and Counseling

Alabama	800-243-5463
Alaska	800-478-6065
Arizona	800-432-4040
Arkansas	800-852-5494
California	800-434-0222
Colorado	800-544-9181
Connecticut	800-994-9422
Delaware	800-336-9500
District of Columbia	202-676-3900
Florida	800-963-5337
Georgia	800-669-8387
Hawaii	808-586-0100
Idaho	800-488-5725
Illinois	800-548-9034
Indiana	800-452-4800
Iowa	800-351-4664
Kansas	800-432-3535
Kentucky	502-564-7372
Louisiana	800-259-5301
Maine	800-750-5353
Maryland	800-243-3425
Massachusetts	800-882-2003

Michigan	800-803-7174
Minnesota	800-882-6262
Mississippi	800-948-3090
Missouri	800-390-3330
Montana	800-332-2272
Nebraska	402-471-2201
Nevada	800-307-4444
New Hampshire	800-852-3388
New Jersey	800-792-8820
New Mexico	800-432-2080
New York	800-333-4114
North Carolina	800-443-9354
North Dakota	800-247-0560
Ohio	800-686-1578
Oklahoma	800-763-2828
Oregon	800-722-4134
Pennsylvania	800-783-7067
Rhode Island	800-322-2880
South Carolina	800-868-9095
South Dakota	605-773-3656
Tennessee	800-525-2816
Texas	800-252-3439
Utah	800-439-3805
Vermont	802-828-2900
Virginia	800-552-3402
Washington	800-605-6299
West Virginia	800-642-9004
Wisconsin	800-242-1060
Wyoming	800-856-4398
Puerto Rico	787-721-5710
Virgin Islands	809-774-7166

SECTION K
Definitions

Actual Charge — The amount that your doctor, lab, or other medical care supplier bills to you. This is not necessarily the same as the amount that Medicare will pay. It is what the supplier or doctor believes the service or care is worth.

Approved Amount — This is the amount that Medicare decides that the medical service or physician's care is worth. It may or may not be the same as the Actual Charge billed. If it is less, you may or may not be responsible for the difference.

Assignment — This is an arrangement between Medicare and your physician or supplier in which s/he agrees to accept as full payment whatever the Medicare Approved Amount is. This is generally beneficial to the patient, although it does not relieve the patient of responsibility for deductibles or co-insurance payments.

Beneficiary — A Medicare Beneficiary is the person who is enrolled in the Medicare program and receives the medical or other related services (i.e., the patient).

Benefit Period — A benefit period is a time frame. Benefit periods have beginnings and endings and affect your costs. They are used to make calculations about deductibles, co-payment amounts, and total covered costs.

Co-insurance — This is the amount of the charge (often a percentage) that the patient is responsible for paying.

Coordination of Benefits — A process agreed to among insurers to prevent a patient being reimbursed for more than 100% when there is more than one insurance company making payment on the same claim.

Co-payment — The amount of money the patient is responsible for paying for a given service.

Deductible — This is the initial amount of money for which the patient is responsible in any specific Benefit Period. There is generally one deductible per Benefit Period.

Diagnosis Related Group (DRG) — A system of payment used by Medicare to reimburse hospitals based on the average costs to treat a particular illness.

Durable Medical Equipment — Medical equipment that is able to be used over a long period of time (e.g., wheelchairs, walkers, hospital beds).

Emergency Care — Medical care required to prevent imminent death, disability or injury.

Excess Charge — The difference between the Medicare Approved Amount and the Actual Charge, when the Actual Charge is more.

Explanation of Medicare Benefits (EOMB) — This is the form which is sent to you which details the dates and services or doctors involved, the expenses which Medicare will allow, what they have paid and to whom, and what your financial responsibility is. This is the first information which you will receive from Medicare about your coverage.

Fee-for-Service — This is the traditional type of medical provider/patient relationship. It means that the patient chooses his/her medical provider and then is billed by that provider a fee for the services rendered. This can be a doctor's fee or any other type of medical service. Under a Fee for Service arrangement, there are no restrictions about who you choose and you do not need to receive prior permission from anyone, unlike in a managed care type of system.

Freedom of Choice Option — An option available in some managed care plans that allows the patient to seek medical services outside the network of doctors and providers.

General Enrollment Period — The period from January 1st to March 31st each year when those eligible can enroll in Part B of Medicare.

Health Care Financing Administration — An agency of the US Department of Health and Human Services which is responsible for running the Medicare program.

Health Maintenance Organization (HMO) — An organization that acts as both the insurer and the provider of care for a prepaid fee. Such organizations generally have a specific group of doctors, specialists and other providers who must be used by the patient in order to obtain benefits.

Home Health Agency — A Medicare approved agency which provides in-home care for eligible patients.

Inpatient — Someone who is actually admitted to a hospital or other medical facility for at least one night. Going to a hospital for a medical procedure, even a surgical one, does not mean you are an "inpatient." You must stay overnight at the recommendation of your physician.

Intermediate Care Facility — A facility that provides less intensive care than a skilled nursing facility, but is more rehabilitative than the custodial care of a nursing home.

Limiting Charge — The calculation that controls the amount that a non-participating doctor is allowed to charge a Medicare patient. It caps the amount above the Medicare approved charge that a doctor can collect from you.

Managed Care — This is a medical care delivery system, such as an HMO or PPO, where someone "manages" your care by making decisions regarding which medical services you can use. Each plan has its own group of hospitals, doctors and other providers and you generally must receive all your care through someone in this network. The benefits of managed care types of plans are that they often cover preventive care and do not usually require you to fill out any paperwork. Depending upon the plan, they may or may not have a co-payment.

Medicaid — A government sponsored and state run program to aid the poor. Within the guidelines set by the federal government, the states control eligibility standards and benefits for medical and other care.

Medically Necessary — Medical services which are accepted as appropriate to the treatment of the patient's condition. Generally, they must be prescribed by a physician.

Medicare — A federal insurance program providing medical benefits to people over age 65, the permanently disabled and people with kidney failure.

Medicare Carrier — These are the organizations (usually insurance companies) which the government uses to process Medicare Part B claims. The information number listed on your

289

EOMB form is that of your Medicare Carrier. The companies vary by state or region and a complete list may be found in Appendix A.

Medicare Hospital Insurance — Part A of Medicare, which covers medically necessary inpatient care in a hospital, skilled nursing facility or psychiatric hospital. It also covers costs related to certain hospice and home health care services.

Medicare Intermediary — These are the organizations which Medicare uses to process Part A claims. A complete list is found in Appendix A.

Medicare Medical Insurance — Part B of Medicare, which covers medically necessary doctor, laboratory, and other medical services which are not covered by Part A. Costs can be incurred in or out of a hospital.

Medicare Part A — The same as Medicare Hospital Insurance.

Medicare Part B — The same as Medicare Medical insurance.

Medicare SELECT — A Medigap policy that requires the use of providers within a specified network.

Medigap Insurance — Insurance policies which supplement the coverage provided by Medicare Part A and Part B benefits.

Nonparticipating Physician — A doctor who does not pledge to accept assignment on all claims by signing the Medicare participation agreement.

Outpatient — A patient who is treated at a hospital or other skilled medical facility without being admitted to the facility overnight.

Out-of-Area Care — Care given to an HMO member outside the area of service for the HMO.

Out-of-Pocket Charges — The amount of money the patient will be responsible for paying for any medical service after all insurance payments have been received.

Participating Physician or Supplier — This is a doctor or supplier who agrees to accept Assignment on all claims. This is helpful in reducing costs to the patient.

Peer Review Organization (PRO) — A group of medical professionals who have the authority to review medical cases and make decisions on behalf of Medicare as to the medical necessity of the treatment. PROs also handle Requests for Reconsideration of Medicare hospital claim denials.

Preferred Provider Organization (PPO) — Similar to an HMO, this type of organization encourages patients to use a specific group of providers. This is usually accomplished by paying a greater portion of the fee if the patient uses someone on the list of approved providers.

Pre-existing Conditions — Medical conditions or illnesses that are in existence before an insurance policy becomes effective.

Primary Care Physician — In a managed care organization, this is the doctor who is primarily responsible for your health care. All your care within the network of providers is controlled by your primary care physician. S/he will refer you to specialists and other providers as s/he deems necessary.

Primary Payer — Generally this is Medicare, and it is the entity that has initial responsibility for the payment of the bill, or the first place that the bill for medical services should be submitted. You may have secondary payers, such as Medigap policies, which will require submittal of the bill after the Primary payer is done with it. Under some circumstances,

291

Medicare is not the primary payer, for example, if you are covered by an employer sponsored health care plan. It is very important to understand who your Primary Payer is, as it affects your paperwork and your reimbursement.

Provider — A person (e.g., a doctor) or a company (e.g., a lab) which is approved to render medical or related services.

Secondary Payer — The party (insurance company or Medicare) who is responsible for payments after the Primary Payer has processed the claim. If you are working and covered by an employer sponsored group health care plan, Medicare will be the secondary payer.

Service Area — The area in which a managed care organization has agreed to provide medical services.

Skilled Nursing Facility — A facility that provides skilled nursing and rehabilitation services. It may or may not be part of a hospital. It not a nursing home.

Utilization Review Committee (URC) — A committee of hospital physicians who review hospital cases and make decisions about appropriate care, admissions, discharges and length of stay.

INDEX

End Stage Renal Disease 53-58

Enrollment 29, 30-39, 41, 42, 43, 59, 121, 141-142, 146, 168, 169, 170, 182

EOMB 17, 21, 23, 80, 89, 92, 93, 94, 99, 100, 101, 102, 113, 114, 116, 118, 207

ESRD *see End Stage Renal Disease*

Excess charge 17, 23

Expedited determination 118, 151

F

Farm worker 45

Federal government worker 26, 29

Fee-for-service 9, 18, 23, 86, 120, 135, 142, 146, 153, 155, 166, 205, 205

Finance 188

Finances 163, 186-199, 200

Financial need 10, 174, 177, 178

Financial resources 8, 10, 178, 179, 186-199, 201, 211

Frequently Asked Questions 11, 21, 40, 59, 80, 98, 116, 134, 152, 160, 170, 178, 184, 197, 205, 215

G

Gaps 10, 122, 134, 146, 186, 188, 190, 194, 204, 218

Government workers 27

H

HCFA *see Health Care Financing Administration*

HCPP 142, 144, 146

Health Care Financing Administration 6-7, 12, 110, 114, 118, 141, 150, 152, 160, 162, 163, 165, 169

Health Maintenance Organization 18, 19, 135, 136, 140, 153, 155, 156, 167, 170, 185, 203

HMO *see Health Maintenance Organization*

Home health care 17, 67, 71-73, 84, 104, 112, 118, 148, 157, 158, 160, 191, 215, 216

Hospice 17, 67, 74-77, 81, 82, 83, 84, 85, 104, 112, 167, 189, 191, 210

I

Intermediate care 69, 194, 195, 198, 210, 212

K

Kidney failure 40, 46, 53-58, 59-61, 142

Kidney transplant 53-58, 61, 142

L

Lifetime reserve days 69, 82, 189, 199

Long term care 10, 13, 68, 148, 187, 188, 198, 200, 203, 207, 208, 210-217

Long term illness 98

Stay up to date on Medicare.

If you would like to keep up on changes to Medicare, fill out the coupon below and return it to us. We'll add you to our free mailing list for information on Medicare.

PLEASE PRINT

Name _____

Address _____

City _____

State _____

Zip _____

Phone _____

E-mail address _____

Mail to:
Department 101
Race Point Press
PO Box 770
Provincetown, MA 02657-0770
or
E-mail the information above to info@RacePointPress.com

If you would like to order a copy of
The Medicare Answer Book, please call
toll-free (888) 446-5544.